Medifocus Guidebook on.

Parkinson's Disease

Last Update: 23 January 2012

Medifocus.com, Inc.

11529 Daffodil Lane
Suite 200
Silver Spring, MD 20902

www.medifocus.com

(800) 965-3002

MediFocus Guide #NR013

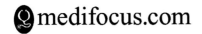medifocus.com

How To Use This Medifocus Guidebook

Before you start to review your *Guidebook*, it would be helpful to familiarize yourself with the organization and content of the information that is included in the Guidebook. Your *MediFocus Guidebook* is organized into the following five major sections.

- **Section 1: Background Information** - This section provides detailed information about the organization and content of the *Guidebook* including tips and suggestions for conducting additional research about the condition.

- **Section 2: The Intelligent Patient Overview** - This section is a comprehensive overview of the condition and includes important information about the cause of the disease, signs and symptoms, how the condition is diagnosed, the treatment options, quality of life issues, and questions to ask your doctor.

- **Section 3: Guide to the Medical Literature** - This section opens the door to the latest cutting-edge research and clinical advances recently published in leading medical journals. It consists of an extensive, focused selection of journal article references with links to the PubMed abstracts (summaries) of the articles. PubMed is the U.S. National Library of Medicine's database of references and abstracts from more than 4,500 medical and scientific articles published worldwide.

- **Section 4: Centers of Research** - This section is a unique directory of doctors, researchers, hospitals, medical centers, and research institutions with specialized interest and, in many cases, clinical expertise in the management of patients with the condition. You can use the "Centers of Research" directory to contact, consults, or network with leading experts in the field and to locate a hospital or medical center that can help you.

- **Section 5: Tips for Finding and Choosing a Doctor** - This section of your *Guidebook* offers important tips for how to find physicians as well as suggestions for how to make informed choices about choosing a doctor who is right for you.

- **Section 6: Directory of Organizations** - This section of your *Guidebook* is a directory of select disease organizations and support groups that are in the business of helping patients and their families by providing access to information, resources, and services. Many of these organizations can answer your questions, enable you to network with other patients, and help you find a doctor in your geographical area who specializes in managing your condition.

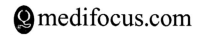

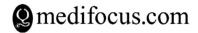
medifocus.com

Disclaimer

Medifocus.com, Inc. serves only as a clearinghouse for medical health information and does not directly or indirectly practice medicine. Any information provided by *Medifocus.com, Inc.* is intended solely for educating our clients and should not be construed as medical advice or guidance, which should always be obtained from a licensed physician or other health-care professional. As such, the client assumes full responsibility for the appropriate use of the medical and health information contained in the Guidebook and agrees to hold *Medifocus.com, Inc.* and any of its third-party providers harmless from any and all claims or actions arising from the clients' use or reliance on the information contained in this Guidebook. Although *Medifocus.com, Inc.* makes every reasonable attempt to conduct a thorough search of the published medical literature, the possibility always exists that some significant articles may be missed.

Copyright

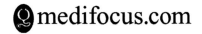

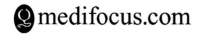medifocus.com

Table of Contents

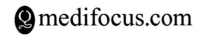

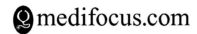
1 - Background Information

Introduction

Chronic or life-threatening illnesses can have a devastating impact on both the patient and the family. In today's new world of medicine, many consumers have come to realize that they are the ones who are primarily responsible for their own health care as well as for the health care of their loved ones.

When facing a chronic or life-threatening illness, you need to become an educated consumer in order to make an informed health care decision. Essentially that means finding out everything about the illness - the treatment options, the doctors, and the hospitals - so that you can become an educated health care consumer and make the tough decisions. In the past, consumers would go to a library and read everything available about a particular illness or medical condition. In today's world, many turn to the Internet for their medical information needs.

The first sites visited are usually the well known health "portals" or disease organizations and support groups which contain a general overview of the condition for the layperson. That's a good start but soon all of the basic information is exhausted and the need for more advanced information still exists. What are the latest "cutting-edge" treatment options? What are the results of the most up-to-date clinical trials? Who are the most notable experts? Where are the top-ranked medical institutions and hospitals?

The best source for authoritative medical information in the United States is the National Library of Medicine's medical database called PubMed, that indexes citations and abstracts (brief summaries) of over 7 million articles from more than 3,800 medical journals published worldwide. PubMed was developed for medical professionals and is the primary source utilized by health care providers for keeping up with the latest advances in clinical medicine.

A typical PubMed search for a specific disease or condition, however, usually retrieves hundreds or even thousands of "hits" of journal article citations. That's an avalanche of information that needs to be evaluated and transformed into truly useful knowledge. What are the most relevant journal articles? Which ones apply to your specific situation? Which articles are considered to be the most authoritative - the ones your physician would rely on in making clinical decisions? This is where *Medifocus.com* provides an effective solution.

Medifocus.com has developed an extensive library of *MediFocus Guidebooks* covering a wide spectrum of chronic and life threatening diseases. Each *MediFocus Guidebook* is a high quality, up- to-date digest of "professional-level" medical information consisting of the most relevant citations and abstracts of journal articles published in authoritative, trustworthy medical journals. This information represents the latest advances known to modern medicine for the treatment and management of the condition, including published results from clinical trials. Each *Guidebook* also includes a valuable index of leading authors and medical institutions as well as a directory of disease organizations and support groups. *MediFocus Guidebooks* are reviewed, revised and updated every 4-months to ensure that you receive the latest and most up-to-date information about the specific condition.

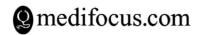medifocus.com

About Your MediFocus Guidebook

Introduction

Your *MediFocus Guidebook* is a valuable resource that represents a comprehensive synthesis of the most up-to-date, advanced medical information published about the condition in well-respected, trustworthy medical journals. It is the same type of professional-level information used by physicians and other health-care professionals to keep abreast of the latest developments in biomedical research and clinical medicine. The *Guidebook* is intended for patients who have a need for more advanced, in-depth medical information than is generally available to consumers from a variety of other resources. The primary goal of a *MediFocus Guidebook* is to educate patients and their families about their treatment options so that they can make informed health-care decisions and become active participants in the medical decision making process.

The *Guidebook* production process involves a team of experienced medical research professionals with vast experience in researching the published medical literature. This team approach to the development and production of the *MediFocus Guidebooks* is designed to ensure the accuracy, completeness, and clinical relevance of the information. The *Guidebook* is intended to serve as a basis for a more meaningful discussion between patients and their health-care providers in a joint effort to seek the most appropriate course of treatment for the disease.

Guidebook Organization and Content

Section 1 - Background Information
This section provides detailed information about the organization and content of the *Guidebook* including tips and suggestions for conducting additional research about the condition.

Section 2 - The Intelligent Patient Overview
This section of your *MediFocus Guidebook* represents a detailed overview of the disease or condition specifically written from the patient's perspective. It is designed to satisfy the basic informational needs of consumers and their families who are confronted with the illness and are facing difficult choices. Important aspects which are addressed in "The Intelligent Patient" section include:

- The etiology or cause of the disease
- Signs and symptoms
- How the condition is diagnosed

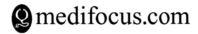
- The current standard of care for the disease
- Treatment options
- New developments
- Important questions to ask your health care provider

Section 3 - Guide to the Medical Literature

This is a roadmap to important and up-to-date medical literature published about the condition from authoritative, trustworthy medical journals. This is the same information that is used by physicians and researchers to keep up with the latest developments and breakthroughs in clinical medicine and biomedical research. A broad spectrum of articles is included in each *MediFocus Guidebook* to provide information about standard treatments, treatment options, new clinical developments, and advances in research. To facilitate your review and analysis of this information, the articles are grouped by specific categories. A typical *MediFocus Guidebook* usually contains one or more of the following article groupings:

- *Review Articles:* Articles included in this category are broad in scope and are intended to provide the reader with a detailed overview of the condition including such important aspects as its cause, diagnosis, treatment, and new advances.

- *General Interest Articles:* These articles are broad in scope and contain supplementary information about the condition that may be of interest to select groups of patients.

- *Drug Therapy:* Articles that provide information about the effectiveness of specific drugs or other biological agents for the treatment of the condition.

- *Surgical Therapy:* Articles that provide information about specific surgical treatments for the condition.

- *Clinical Trials:* Articles in this category summarize studies which compare the safety and efficacy of a new, experimental treatment modality to currently available standard treatments for the condition. In many cases, clinical trials represent the latest advances in the field and may be considered as being on the "cutting edge" of medicine. Some of these experimental treatments may have already been incorporated into clinical practice.

The following information is provided for each of the articles referenced in this section of your *MediFocus Guidebook:*

- Article title

medifocus.com

- Author Name(s)
- Institution where the study was done
- Journal reference (Volume, page numbers, year of publication)
- Link to Abstract (brief summary of the actual article)

Linking to Abstracts: Most of the medical journal articles referenced in this section of your *MediFocus Guidebook* include an abstract (brief summary of the actual article) that can be accessed online via the National Library of Medicine's PubMed® database. You can easily access the individual article abstracts online by entering the individual URL address for a particular article into your web browser, or by going to the URL listed on the bottom of each page of this section.

Section 4 - Centers of Research

We've compiled a unique directory of doctors, researchers, medical centers, and research institutions with specialized research interest, and in many cases, clinical expertise in the management of the specific medical condition. The "Centers of Research" directory is a valuable resource for quickly identifying and locating leading medical authorities and medical institutions within the United States and other countries that are considered to be at the forefront in clinical research and treatment of the condition.

Inclusion of the names of specific doctors, researchers, hospitals, medical centers, or research institutions in this *Guidebook* does not imply endorsement by Medifocus.com, Inc. or any of its affiliates. Consumers are encouraged to conduct additional research to identify health-care professionals, hospitals, and medical institutions with expertise in providing specific medical advice, guidance, and treatment for this condition.

Section 5 - Tips on Finding and Choosing a Doctor

One of the most important decisions confronting patients who have been diagnosed with a serious medical condition is finding and choosing a qualified physician who will deliver high-level, quality medical care in accordance with curently accepted guidelines and standards of care. Finding the "best" doctor to manage your condition, however, can be a frustrating and time-consuming experience unless you know what you are looking for and how to go about finding it. This section of your Guidebook offers important tips for how to find physicians as well as suggestions for how to make informed choices about choosing a doctor who is right for you.

Section 6 - Directory of Organizations

This section of your *Guidebook* is a directory of select disease organizations and support groups that are in the business of helping patients and their families by providing access to information, resources, and services. Many of these organizations can answer your questions, enable you to network with other patients, and help you find a doctor in your

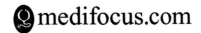

geographical area who specializes in managing your condition.

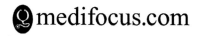medifocus.com

Ordering Full-Text Articles

After reviewing your *MediFocus Guidebook*, you may wish to order the full-text copy of some of the journal article citations that are referenced in the *Guidebook*. There are several options available for obtaining full-text copies of journal articles, however, with the exception of obtaining the article yourself by visiting a nearby medical library, most involve a fee to cover the costs of photocopying, delivering, and paying the copyright royalty fees set by the individual publishers of medical journals.

This section of your *MediFocus Guidebook* provides some basic information about how you can go about obtaining full-text copies of journal articles from various fee-based document delivery resources.

Commercial Document Delivery Services

There are numerous commercial document delivery companies that provide full-text photocopying and delivery services to the general public. The costs may vary from company to company so it is worth your while to carefully shop-around and compare prices. Some of these commercial document delivery services enable you to order articles directly online from the company's web site. You can locate companies that provide document delivery services by typing the key words "document delivery" into any major Internet search engine.

National Library of Medicine's "Loansome Doc" Document Retrieval Services

The National Library of Medicine (NLM), located in Bethesda, Maryland, offers full-text photocopying and delivery of journal articles through its on-line service known as "Loansome Doc". To learn more about how you can order articles using "Loansome Doc", please visit the NLM web site at:
http://www.nlm.nih.gov/pubs/factsheets/loansome_doc.html

Participating "Loansome Doc" Libraries: United States

In the United States there are approximately 250 medical libraries that participate in the National Library of Medicine's "Loansome Doc" document retrieval and delivery services for the general public. Please note that each participating library sets its own policies and

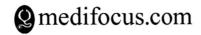

charges for providing document retrieval services. To order full-text copies of articles, simply contact a participating "Loansome Doc" medical library in your geographical area and ask to speak with one of the reference librarians. They can answer all of your questions including fees, delivery options, and turn-around time.

Here is how to find a participating "Loansome Doc" library in the U.S. that provides article retrieval services for the general public:

- **United States** - Contact a Regional Medical Library at 1-800-338-7657 (Monday - Friday; 8:30 AM - 5:30 PM). They will provide information about libraries in your area with which you may establish an account for the "Loansome Doc" service.

- **Canada** - Contact the Canada Institute for Scientific and Technical Information (CISTI) at 1-800-668-1222 for information about libraries in your area.

International MEDLARS Centers

If you reside outside the United States, you can obtain copies of medical journal articles through one of several participating International Medical Literature Analysis and Retrieval Systems (MEDLARS) Centers that provide "Loansome Doc" services in over 20 major countries. International MEDLARS Centers can be found in some of these countries: Australia, Canada, China, Egypt, France, Germany, Hong Kong, India, Israel, Italy, Japan, Korea, Kuwait, Mexico, Norway, Russia, South Africa, Sweden, and the United Kingdom. A complete listing of International MEDLARS Centers, including locations and telephone contact information can be viewed at:
http://www.nlm.nih.gov/pubs/factsheets/intlmedlars.html

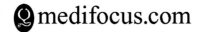

NOTES

Use this page for taking notes as you review your Guidebook

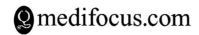

2 - The Intelligent Patient Overview

PARKINSON'S DISEASE

Introduction to Parkinson's Disease

Parkinson's disease is a progressive, neurodegenerative disorder that affects movement, muscle control, and balance as well as numerous other functions. It is part of a group of conditions known as *motor systems disorders*. Parkinson's disease was named for James Parkinson, a general practitioner in London during the 19th century who first described the symptoms of the disease. Symptoms describing Parkinson's disease are mentioned in the writings of medicine in India dating back to 5,000 BCE as well as in Chinese writings dating back approximately 2500 years. Parkinson's disease is the most common movement disorder and the second most common neurodegenerative disorder, the most common being Alzheimer's disease.

The hallmark symptoms of Parkinson's disease (PD) are asymmetric tremors at rest, rigidity, and *bradykinesia* (slowness in movement). There is currently no cure for Parkinson's disease; it is always chronic and progressive, meaning that the symptoms always exist and always worsen over time. The rate of progression varies from person to person, as does the intensity of the symptoms. Parkinson's disease itself is not a fatal disease and many people live into their older years. Mortality of Parkinson's disease patients is usually related to secondary complications, such as pneumonia or falling-related injuries.

There are three types of Parkinson's disease and they are grouped by age of onset:

- *Adult-Onset Parkinson's Disease* - This is the most common type of Parkinson's disease. The average age of onset is approximately 60 years old. The incidence of adult onset PD rises noticeably as people advance in age into their 70's and 80's.

- *Young-Onset Parkinson's Disease* - The age of onset is between 21-40 years old. Though the incidence of Young-Onset Parkinson's Disease is very high in Japan (approximately 40% of cases diagnosed with Parkinson's disease), it is still relatively uncommon in the U.S., with estimates ranging from 5-10% of cases diagnosed.

- *Juvenile Parkinson's Disease* - The age of onset is before the age of 21. The

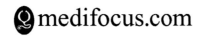

incidence of Juvenile Parkinson's Disease is very rare.

Parkinson's disease can significantly impair quality of life not only for the patients but for their families as well, and especially for the primary caregivers. It is therefore important for caregivers and family members to educate themselves and become familiar with the course of Parkinson's disease and the progression of symptoms so that they can be actively involved in communication with health care providers and in understanding all decisions regarding treatment of the patient.

Epidemiology of Parkinson's Disease

According to the American Parkinson's Disease Association, there are approximately 1.5 million people in the U.S. who suffer from Parkinson's disease - approximately 1-2% of people over the age of 60 and 3-5% of the population over age 85. The incidence of PD ranges from 8.6-19 per 100,000 people. Approximately 50,000 new cases are diagnosed in the U.S. annually. That number is expected to rise as the general population in the U.S. ages. Onset of Parkinson's disease before the age of 40 is rare. All races and ethnic groups are affected.

The incidence of Parkinson's disease among males and females is generally equally distributed when onset of disease is before the age of 60. When onset is past 60 years of age, most studies report a higher incidence in males.

Pathophysiology of Parkinson's Disease

Deep in the brain, below the cerebral cortex, there are interconnected areas of grey matter collectively known as the *basal ganglia* (literally "basement structures"). These structures include the *caudate nucleus*, *putamen*, and *globus pallidum internus* (GPi) which are involved in controlling voluntary movement. The nerve cells in the *substantia nigra* (a cluster of cells located next to the basal ganglia) produce *dopamine*, an essential neurotransmitter that is responsible for transmitting electrical signals between nerve cells. The substantia nigra sends out fibers to the *corpus striatum* (grey and white bands of tissue in the caudate nucleus and putamen) where the dopamine is released. The transmission of dopamine and its release into the corpus striatum is necessary for smooth, coordinated muscle movement.

Parkinson's disease occurs when there is a disruption of dopamine production which leads to impaired neurotransmission (communication between brain cells) in the basal ganglia. The reduced level of dopamine causes the nerve cells to fire out of control and causes a loss of smooth, controlled muscle activity. The death of dopamine-producing cells in the substantia nigra, resulting in a reduced level of dopamine in the corpus striatum, is the primary pathology in Parkinson's disease. By the time symptoms develop, there is at least a 60% loss of dopamine-producing cells in the substantia nigra and an 80-90% loss of dopamine in the corpus striatum.

Parkinson's disease is also characterized by the presence of *Lewy bodies*, structures that are found in the cells of the substantia nigra as well as in other secondary locations. Lewy bodies are strongly correlated with neurodegeneration and are considered a diagnostic hallmark of Parkinson's disease.

Increasing evidence suggests that Parkinson's disease is a multi-system brain disease in which various neurotransmitter systems are affected and related deficits become more prominent over the course of the disease. In addition, it is known that the disease process of PD begins long before motor symptoms are clinically visible. Many patients report that they already experienced non-motor symptoms associated with PD, such as fatigue, constipation, and olfactory changes, several years before clinical onset.

Causes of Parkinson's Disease

Researchers have been unable to identify specific causes of Parkinson's disease but there are many theories regarding factors which may individually or in combination play a role in its development. These include:

- Genetics - Researchers have found gene mutations related to juvenile and early-onset PD. Recently, a new mutation was identified on the LRRK2 gene that is believed to be related to idiopathic PD.

- Family history - According to the National Institute of Neurologic Disorders and Stroke (NINDS) approximately 15-20% of patients with Parkinson's disease have a close relative who exhibited a parkinsonian symptom. Estimates are that the risk for developing PD for family members of a patient with PD is 3-4 times that of the general population. There is a theory that if the right factors come together in an individual with a predisposition based on family history, that individual will develop Parkinson's disease.

- Oxidative damage - Free radicals (unstable molecules) circulating in the brain may cause oxidation resulting in damage to neurons. Some researchers refer to free radicals as endogenous toxins (toxins produced by the body).

- Toxins - Exposure to environmental toxins such as pesticides may cause degeneration of the dopamine producing cells. It is known that exposure to the herbicide Paraquat elevates the risk for PD. Although not clearly understood, it appears that smoking lowers the risk of developing PD.

- Occupational exposure - There is a higher prevalence in certain occupations such as welders, farmers, cabinet makers, and cleaners. In addition, drinking well water and industrial exposure to heavy metals (such as iron, zinc, copper, mercury, and magnesium) also elevate the risk of PD.

- Accelerated aging of neural cells - This theory proposes that for unknown reasons, the normal age-related death of brain cells is accelerated in patients with Parkinson's disease, causing the dopamine-producing cells to "age" and die faster than normal.

Parkinson's Disease Rating Scale

Evaluation of motor severity and disability in Parkinson's disease (PD) is important as it is the only way available to chart the course of disease progression in each patient and to document the outcome of rehabilitation. The progression of Parkinson's disease is usually documented using the Unified Parkinson Disease Rating Scale (UPDRS), a rating scale introduced in 1987. There are three sections of the UPDRS which evaluate the major areas of disability in Parkinson's disease and one that evaluates complications of treatment and they include:

- Cognition, behavior, mood

  - intellectual impairment
  - thought disorder
  - motivation/initiative
  - depression

- Activities of daily living

  - speech
  - salivation
  - swallowing
  - handwriting
  - cutting food
  - dressing
  - hygiene
  - turning in bed
  - falling

- freezing
- walking
- tremor
- sensory complaints

- Motor abilities

  - speech
  - facial expression
  - tremor at rest
  - action tremor
  - rigidity
  - finger taps
  - hand movements
  - hand pronation (rotation of the hands and forearms so that the palms face downward)
  - supination (rotation of the hands and forearms so that the palms face upward)
  - leg agility
  - arising from chair
  - posture
  - gait
  - postural stability
  - body bradykinesia (slow movement)

- Complications of treatment

  - dyskinesia (difficulty in performing voluntary movements) including duration, level of disability, and pain
  - early morning dystonia (twisting and repetitive movements or abnormal postures)
  - "off-period" deterioration (period between two scheduled doses of levodopa when disease symptoms such as tremors, rigidity, and bradykinesia are more intense) including the *duration* of the "off" period, predictability based on dose, and the pattern of onset (sudden or gradual)
  - anorexia (including nausea and/or vomiting)
  - sleep disturbance
  - symptomatic orthostasis (difficulty remaining upright, typically due to a drop in blood pressure)

The scale is administered by a health professional and points are assigned to each item based on patient response and physical examination. Parts I, II, and III contain 44 questions and each is measured on a 5-point scale, while part IV contains 11 questions and the scale can range from 0 to 23. The cumulative score ranges from 0 (no disability) to 199 (total disability).

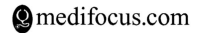

Diagnosis of Parkinson's Disease

Signs and Symptoms of Parkinson's Disease

Early presentation of Parkinson's disease (PD) is often missed because the symptoms can be subtle and the progression of disease is typically slow. A patient may complain of generally not feeling well, or feeling a little down, or just a little shaky. Usually, it is friends or family who first notice that something may be wrong and they will encourage the individual to be seen by a doctor.

There are four primary symptoms of Parkinson's disease, known as *TRAP*:

- Tremor
- Rigidity
- Akinesia and Bradykinesia
- Postural Instability

Tremor

Most patients with PD present with a tremor on one side (*unilateral* or *asymmetric*) which is more noticeable at rest. Most often the tremor is noticeable in one hand with the typical "pill-rolling" movement of the thumb and opposing fingers. Tremor can also occur in the tongue, lower jaw, or legs. Some patients report a feeling of internal shaking which is not visible to others. A resting tremor is present in 70-80% of people diagnosed with Parkinson's disease and disappears with action of the hand. It is also frequently noticeable when the patient is walking.

Tremor is often the primary symptom which spurs a patient to seek medical help since it is so noticeable and can also interfere with daily activities. Severity varies among patients but tremors almost always worsen with fatigue, stress, anxiety, excitement, apprehension, and cold weather. Tremors usually disappear during sleep. In older adults, tremors are less common. Approximately 25% of patients do not develop tremors.

Rigidity

Rigidity consists of increased tone or stiffness of the muscles. Most patients with early Parkinson's disease do not report a feeling of rigidity but may report feelings of vague aching or discomfort in a limb. However, when the physician manipulates the limb during the physical examination, signs of rigidity become evident. There is resistance to passive movement which may be seen at any point in testing the full range of motion of the affected limb. If a tremor exists in the rigid limb, one may see smooth movement replaced with a broken up ratchet-type of action ("cogwheel rigidity").

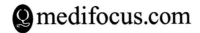

When rigidity occurs in the face, it can cause the classic "mask-like" appearance associated with Parkinson's disease. Rigidity can occur in any limb, the neck, or facial musculature. Some patients report pain due to the rigidity of arms and shoulders. Rigidity is not a part of the normal aging process, so if an individual presents to a doctor with rigidity and improves with anti-parkinsonian drugs, it is most likely caused by Parkinson's disease. Rigidity is not as common a symptom as tremor in patients with Parkinson's disease.

Akinesia and Bradykinesia

Akinesia_ refers to a significant reduction or absence of spontaneous movement and *bradykinesia* refers to slowness of movement. Bradykinesia occurs frequently in PD and affects fine motor and gross motor function. It is usually reported to be the most distressing and troubling symptom as it makes the simplest of tasks very time consuming. It is manifested in a delay of movement initiation (e.g., taking the first step in walking) and slow response once the action begins (e.g., walking very slowly). Bradykinesia interferes with many daily activities such as walking, dressing, household chores, and getting up from or sitting down in a chair.

An especially frustrating aspect of bradykinesia is that it is unpredictable and can occur in the middle of an activity. Two of the most common aspects of Parkinson's-related bradykinesia are that it is usually *asymmetric*, occurring on only one side (in up to 75% of patients) and that fatigue sets in with continued activity. This can be seen when a patient is asked to tap the thumb and index finger together rapidly. Typically, the rate of tapping progressively slows down in the PD patient.

In addition to affecting fine and gross motor function, bradykinesia also affects repetitive movement. Thus, the patient notices difficulty in activities that require dexterity such as fastening buttons, or in tasks requiring repetitive hand motions such as brushing teeth.

In the face, bradykinesia may manifest itself as a decrease in facial expression and/or eye blinking. Some patients experience slowness in the muscles involved in swallowing, leading to a buildup of saliva which could cause choking.

Postural Instability

Postural instability is a general term that involves gait changes and an impaired sense of balance. It is one of the *axial* (spine-related) symptoms of PD that involve the head and trunk, rather than the limbs. Postural instability is noticeable when individuals with PD move or turn abruptly which may cause them to lose their balance and fall. Gait changes include asymmetric slowness, shuffling, and reduced arm swinging. Some individuals with PD lean forward or backward, also causing them to fall easily especially if they are bumped. For some patients, especially older adults, postural instability may be a later

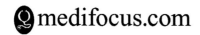

presenting symptom of Parkinson's disease.

Various studies have shown that:

- In a group of PD patients without dementia that was followed to track the existence and progression of postural instability and gait disturbance, 53% of the patients showed signs of postural instability at the beginning of the study, increasing to 88% at an eight-year follow-up.
- Nearly 70% of patients with PD fall at least once a year.
- The average time from onset of PD until the first fall is approximately nine years.
- The greatest predictor of falling is having fallen in the previous year, not disease severity.

To read more about postural instability and gait disturbances in PD, please click on the following link: http://www.ncbi.nlm.nih.gov/pubmed/18787879

Progression of Parkinson's Disease

As Parkinson's disease progresses beyond the early stage described above, many of the difficulties experienced by patients are related to complications and increasing severity of the four basic categories of symptoms (TRAP), including:

- Difficulty Walking - Problems with walking can occur early or late in Parkinson's disease and include:

  - *festination* - an involuntary tendency to take small shuffling steps or "running steps" resulting in the patient walking with increasing speed to prevent falling. It is related to the abnormal center of gravity experienced by the patient and is sometimes called a "catch-up" gait. Festination consists of a combination of shortening of the stride while quickening the gait. It is often difficult for the patient who is "running" to stop when they reach their destination.

  - lack of arm swinging of one or both arms - this contributes to difficulty walking since the brain associates walking and arm swinging together so that when one is impaired, the other may be impaired as well.

  - stooped posture - this results from a greater contraction of chest muscles than back muscles. Exercise is very important to counteract tightening and muscle contraction since stooped posture affects balance, can interfere with walking, and can result in falling and ensuing injury.

- "freezing" is a sudden, temporary inability to move one's legs or feet. It may present as a sudden inability to initiate movement or to continue walking and often occurs when the PD patient approaches a doorway while walking, turns, or is in an area with many people. Freezing is usually associated with visual cues such as narrow doorways or spaces. It occurs during the "off" period when the effect of medication has worn off and before the next dose takes effect. Freezing appears without warning and can last for several seconds. The duration and frequency of freezing episodes typically increase with the severity of PD. Freezing is one of the major causes of falling in patients with Parkinson's disease and occurs in approximately 30% of cases. Patients with early PD do not experience freezing as frequently as those in later stages of the disease. Risk factors for gait freezing include absence of tremor and longer disease duration. Freezing is strongly associated with other axial (spine-related) symptoms such as postural instability. Anxiety can also play a role in initiating freezing or in preventing its resolution.

- Problems with chewing and swallowing - chewing and swallowing problems relate to the overall symptoms of muscle rigidity and are caused by:

  - tongue - the tongue does not depress sufficiently to allow food to proceed to the throat.
  - throat - bits of food that are not completely swallowed collect in the throat and may fall into the airway causing coughing or choking.
  - esophagus - muscles in the gastrointestinal tract, including the muscles involved with moving food down into the stomach from the esophagus, can be affected by PD resulting in food chunks feeling like they are "stuck" or going down slowly. This can lead to heartburn or gastroesophageal reflux.

- Drooling - Excessive drooling occurs when saliva accumulates at the back of the mouth and because of impaired musculature, is not swallowed. In addition to the embarrassment experienced by the patient, drooling can also be dangerous since it can lead to aspiration of saliva into the lungs and cause choking or pneumonia.

- Loss of automatic movement (e.g., blinking) resulting in a "mask-like" appearance to the face.

- Speech impairment - speech problems include: soft voice, slurring words, speaking too quickly, or hesitating before speaking. Speech impairment may be one of the first presenting symptoms of PD.

- Micrographia (progressively smaller handwriting) - this can appear at any stage

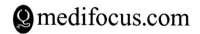

though it often begins to develop before other symptoms of Parkinson's disease are noticeable.

The progression of symptoms in young-onset PD tends to be slower than for adult-onset PD. In addition, symptoms of young-onset PD, such as rigidity, bradykinesia, and dystonia (involuntary muscle spasms, often painful) usually begin symmetrically in the feet, whereas the first symptoms of adult-onset PD are usually asymmetrical (occurring only on one side).

Non-motor Complications of Parkinson's Disease

Parkinson's disease worsens over time and, as the disease progresses so do the complications. Estimates are that up to 80% of people with Parkinson's disease (PD) experience non-motor problems that increase with progression of the disease. These complications become more and more disruptive in the tasks of daily life of and impact significantly on the individual's quality of life. It is important for patients to be made aware of complications that may be anticipated and understand what to expect over the course of the disease. Increasing evidence is pointing to the probability that non-motor features of PD may precede the appearance of motor symptoms by up to several years and, indeed, many patients report experiencing symptoms such as fatigue, depression, constipation, and olfactory changes many years before they are diagnosed with PD.

Non-motor conditions associated with Parkinson's disease may include:

- Cognitive impairment
- Dementia
- Psychosis
- Depression
- Fatigue
- Sleep disturbances
- Disturbances of the autonomic nervous system
- Pain
- Sexual dysfunction
- Emotional disturbances
- Weight loss
- Shortness of breath
- Visual disturbances
- Progressive postural imbalance

Cognitive Impairment

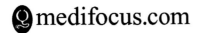

Cognitive impairment is highly variable and may start early in the disease process for some patients with PD, while others may notice changes much later. Studies show that when diagnosed with PD, up to 35% of patients may have signs of cognitive impairment and up to 57% may experience cognitive impairment three years after diagnosis. Cognitive impairment is progressive in severity and the range of deficits becomes wider as injury to cortical tissue spreads. One study reported that 17 years after diagnosis, only 15% of surviving subjects was not cognitively impaired. Some of the functions affected by cognitive impairment include:

- Executive function (the ability to organize cognitive processes such as planning ahead, prioritizing, or shifting from one activity to another)
- Working memory
- Attention
- Visual-spatial dysfunction

Cognitive impairment is related to and impacts many other types of non-motor complications such as dementia, psychosis, depression, apathy, and fatigue.

Dementia

Dementia, a steady, progressive decline in memory and other cognitive functions, is considerably more severe than cognitive impairment and is estimated to occur in approximately 40% of patients diagnosed with Parkinson's disease. One study published in 2003 in *Archives of Neurology* (vol. 60:pp. 387-392) showed that 17 years after diagnosis, approximately 78% of the subjects in the study had dementia. The greatest risk factor for development of dementia in PD is advancing age, not the age of onset, and estimates are that by 90 years of age, 80-90% of PD patients have dementia. The severity of dementia increases as additional cortical structures become affected by the progression of PD. Other risk factors may include: presence of mild cognitive impairment, severity of PD, postural instability, gait disturbance, and speech problems. The risk of a patient with PD developing dementia is six times higher than that of the general population. It is estimated that 3-4% of people with dementia have PD.

A different medical condition known as *dementia with Lewy bodies* presents with dementia and parkinsonian features. It is distinguished from Parkinson's disease by the presence of other associated clinical features (cognitive fluctuations and visual hallucinations) and the temporal course (progression over time). In dementia with Lewy bodies, the interval between the onset of parkinsonian symptoms and dementia is one to two years, while dementia associated with Parkinson's disease typically occurs ten years or more after the onset of Parkinson's disease.

Psychosis

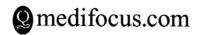

Psychotic symptoms include:

- Illusions - including auditory, olfactory, or tactile (i.e., hearing, smelling, or feeling things that are not real)
- Hallucinations - can be simple or complex, and rarely occur before the initiation of dopaminergic drug treatment and are therefore believed to be closely linked to medication. Additional risk factors for hallucinations may include:

  - duration of PD
  - severity of PD
  - advanced age
  - cognitive impairment
  - visual disorders

- Delusions - beliefs that are not consistent with reality and related to hallucinations (e.g., that a visiting relative is an imposter)

Psychotic symptoms are one of the most common causes for hospitalization of PD patients and for placement in nursing home facilities.

Depression

Depression in Parkinson's disease is relatively common and may occur months or years before other motor-related symptoms are apparent. Up to 20% of patients with PD report having had depressive symptoms even many years before the condition was diagnosed. The risk of depressed people later developing PD is said to be 2-3 times higher than non-depressed people. Various studies have placed the incidence of depression among PD patients at between 12-90%, depending on patient inclusion and criteria for diagnosis of depression. Depression may also be related to chronic pain which affects many people with PD.

The diagnosis of depression can be elusive since symptoms of classic depression (not related to Parkinson's disease) may overlap with symptoms of Parkinson's disease (e.g., mask-face, fatigue, low energy levels). Many symptoms of depression also overlap with symptoms of hypothyroidism (e.g., akinesia, mask-face, mood variations) which affects some Parkinson's disease patients. Depression can also appear as a side effect of some Parkinson's disease medications. It is generally believed that in most PD patients, the severity of depression is mild to moderate, but in patients with dementia, the severity of depression is notably greater. Suicide is typically not associated with depression in PD.

There is increasing evidence that depression is part of the disease process of Parkinson's disease. The reduced dopamine level found in Parkinson's disease patients affects the

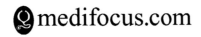medifocus.com

balance of several other neurotransmitters in the brain including *serotonin* which plays a role in depression.

The symptoms of depression in Parkinson's disease include:

- Depressed mood
- Fatigue
- Reduced energy levels
- Reduced appetite
- Sleep disturbances
- Memory disturbances

Doctors should be especially mindful to probe further into the possibility of depression if the patient complains of fatigue and reduced energy levels.

Depression is one of the most prominent non-motor features of Parkinson's disease and is associated with faster progression of motor symptoms, more rapid decline in cognitive function, poorer compliance with Parkinson's medications, and more difficulties in performing routine activities of daily living.

Diagnosing depression in people with Parkinson's disease is sometimes difficult since symptoms of depression may overlap with with those of Parkinson's or other ailments. Treating depression can often help people with Parkinson's disease cope better with the condition and can also improve their quality of life. The two most commonly used classes of prescription medications that are used to manage depression in people with Parkinson's disease are *tricyclic antidepressants* and *selective serotonin reuptake inhibitors* (SSRI's). Although both classes of medications are commonly prescribed by both neurologists and psychiatrists to manage depression in patients with Parkinson's disease, currently there is a lack of sufficient evidence based on randomized clinical trials to recommend one class of medication over the other.

In an article published in the March 10, 2009 issue of *Neurology* (Volume 72; pp. 886-892), researchers from the Robert Wood Johnson Medical School in New Jersey reported the results of a randomized, controlled clinical trial comparing the effectiveness of an antidepressant medication (nortriptyline) to an SSRI (paroxetine CR) in patients with Parkinson's disease. The study included 52 patients with Parkinson's disease who also suffered from depression who were randomly assigned to one of the following treatment groups:

- Nortriptyline - 17 patients received nortriptyline, started at at dose of 25 mg and increased, as needed, upt to 75 mg over 8 weeks.
- Paroxetine CR - 18 patients received paroxetine CR, started at a dose of 12.5 mg that

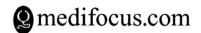

could be increased, as needed, up to 37.5 mg over 8 weeks.
- Placebo - 17 patients received placebo pills, started at 1 pill a day and increased to 3 pills per day.

The study population consisted of 27 men and 25 women with a mean age of 63 years. The mean duration of Parkinson's disease was 6.6 years. Fifty of the patients had major depression while 2 patients had only *dysthymia* (mild but chronic depression). The primary outcome evaluated in this study was an improvement in depression from baseline (before treatment) as measured using the Hamilton Depression Rating Scale and the percentage (%) of subjects in each group who responded to the treatments.

The researchers reported the following major findings from their study:

- Compared to placebo, patients who received nortriptyline experienced a significant reduction in depression as measured with the Hamilton Depression Rating Scale.
- Compared to placebo, no significant reduction in the level of depression was observed for those patients who had received paroxetine CR.
- A head-to-head statistical comparison of nortriptyline versus paroxetine CR showed that a significantly higher number of patients in the nortriptyline group (53%) experienced a 50% or greater reduction in their level of depression as compared to those treated with paroxetine CR.
- Test subjects receiving nortriptyline also reported significant improvements in sleep, anxiety, and social functioning compared to those treated with paroxetine CR.

This is the largest study to date comparing the efficacy of a tricyclic antidepressant (nortriptyline) to an SSRI (paroxetine CR) for the treatment of depression in patients with Parkinson's disease. Although the results of this study suggest that tricyclic antidepressants may be a better choice than SSRI's for the management of depression in Parkinson's disease, the authors of the study noted that additional studies are necessary involving a larger number of patients before more definitive guidelines can be formulated for the clinical treatment of depression in people with Parkinson's disease.

Fatigue

Fatigue in PD includes an overwhelming sense of tiredness and lack of energy that may occur in up to 75% of patients. It appears to intensify as PD progresses, particularly in the presence of depression. Understandably, fatigue has a strong negative impact on quality of life as well as cognitive and physical functioning. Some patients report feeling strong fatigue many years before the clinical onset of PD.

Sleep Disturbances

Sleep disturbances affect up to 70% of Parkinson's disease patients at varying stages of the disease and with varying intensity. There are several types of sleep-related problems, most of which arise either as a result of pathological changes in the brain such as cell loss around arousal centers or as side effects of medication used for treating PD. Sleep disturbances include:

- Insomnia - patients may have no trouble falling asleep but have difficulty staying asleep at night and cannot fall back asleep if they wake up during the night. They also tend to wake up very early in the morning experiencing tremors or feeling very stiff due to the "wearing-off" effect of dopamine-based medication. It is estimated that up to 60% of patients with PD experience insomnia at nine years after onset. One study reported that insomnia was associated with female gender, disease duration, and depressive symptoms.

- Excessive daytime sleepiness (EDS) - this appears to be an independent problem and not a result of fatigue or nighttime insomnia. It is thought to occur in up to 15% of patients nine years after PD onset but other estimates are that 40% of patients may be affected. It is very disruptive and has a strong negative impact on quality of life since it affects many daily activities such as driving, reading, or socializing. The patient may take frequent naps during the day often leading to added difficulty sleeping at night. One study reported EDS to be associated with age, gender (male), use of dopamine-agonist medication, and disease severity.

- REM (rapid eye movement) sleep disorder - the patient physically acts out the dreams that occur during the REM stage of sleep (also called *parasomnia*). This can manifest itself as vocalizations, kicking, trying to choke another person, trying to move as if running, or striking out, thereby potentially causing injury to a spouse or caregiver sitting or sleeping next to them. REM sleep disorder is thought to be due to a lack of the normal inhibition of motor movement during REM sleep. Parkinson's disease patients with this sleep disorder are at increased risk of developing dementia with Lewy bodies later in the course of PD. Up to one-third of PD patients are affected by REM sleep disorder. The incidence of REM sleep disorder is associated with male gender, lower disease severity, and higher doses of levodopa medication. It is thought by some clinicians that REM sleep disorder may be another condition that occurs in many people several years before they are diagnosed with PD and that up to 60% of people who exhibit REM sleep disorder may later develop PD.

- Restless leg syndrome (RLS) - the individual feels the need to move their legs continuously at night to the point of strongly impacting sleep quality. It affects approximately 8-10% of all people over the age of 65. Some studies have shown that RLS may be present in 20-50% of patients with PD but estimates vary widely.

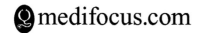

Disturbances of the Autonomic Nervous System

The autonomic nervous system controls involuntary or unconscious body functions such as blood pressure, heart rate, temperature regulation (sweating), and gastrointestinal processes. Autonomic disturbances are increasingly recognized as PD-associated symptoms. Disturbances are associated with increased disease severity, higher doses of dopaminergic medication, and advanced age. Examples of autonomic nervous system disturbances in patients with Parkinson's disease include:

- Constipation - this is common among Parkinson's disease patients since gastrointestinal function slows considerably. It has been reported to predate the onset of PD in many patients by several years. Constipation could also be a side effect of PD medication. Constipation is thought to occur in up to 60% of patients with PD.
- Frequent urination - the bladder senses fullness and contracts prematurely resulting in the patient experiencing a frequent urge to empty the bladder during the day or night.
- Drop of blood pressure with positional change (*orthostatic hypotension*).
- Skin problems - excessively dry or oily skin especially on the face and scalp; reduction of sweating; or episodes of drenching sweats.
- Many PD patients report a loss or reduction in their sense of smell, including odor detection, odor differentiation, and odor identification that may start years before the diagnosis of PD. Odor dysfunction is persistent and not affected by medication. Researchers are investigating the possibility that odor dysfunction may be due to a lesion in the olfactory tract in the brain and may place individuals with idiopathic hyposomnia (reduced smell due to an unknown cause) at a higher risk for PD later in life.
- Hypersalivation - an overproduction of saliva that results in drooling.

Pain

It is estimated that more than half of patients with PD experience pain or discomfort and some of those patients report that their pain is their most significant problem. The Parkinson's Disease Foundation (PDF) report that there are several sources of pain in PD including:

- Musculoskeletal pain - this includes pain related to rigidity, lack of movement, mechanical stresses on the muscles due to postural abnormalities, shoulder stiffness ("frozen shoulder") and contractures due to immobility of a limb. Pain in the hip, back, or neck is common.
- Neuritic pain - this pain occurs close to a nerve or nerve root and is associated with arthritis. A common location is the L-5 lumbar root which causes sciatica.
- Dystonia - pain from dystonia spasms which causes severe, prolonged body twisting and postures, causes the most severe pain for many patients with PD. The spasms

may affect the limbs, trunk, neck, face, tongue, jaw, swallowing muscles, and vocal chords. In addition, it may cause the toes to curl painfully, the arm to pull behind the back, or force the head forward towards the chest. In some patients, dystonia may be related to "wearing off" of medication or may be most severe in the morning when they get up.

- Akathesia - extreme restlessness; this is a severe form of discomfort felt by many patients with PD. They cannot stay still and it severely impacts quality of life since it is literally disabling. Patients may not be able to sit still, lie in bed, drive a car, or remain socially active. If it occurs at night they may lose sleep. The PDF estimates that akathisia is related to medication in approximately 50% of cases.
- Central pain - this is thought to be directly related to PD itself and is described as bizarre sensations such as stabbing or burning pain that may occur anywhere in the body including the abdomen, chest, mouth, rectum, and genitalia.

Sexual Dysfunction

According to the National Parkinson's Foundation, approximately 81% of men and 43% of women report reduced sexual activity with increasing severity of Parkinson's disease. Many men report sexual dissatisfaction because of erectile dysfunction which is thought to affect approximately 30-60% of male PD patients. Sexual dissatisfaction in women is related to the quality of their sexual experiences, poor body image, vaginal tightness, and urinary difficulties such as an increased urge to urinate or urinary incontinence.

Emotional Disturbances

The patient with Parkinson's disease may become anxious, fearful, irritable, lose motivation, or become uncharacteristically pessimistic.

Weight Loss

Weight loss is a significant problem for patients with Parkinson's disease and is related to reduced calorie intake caused by:

- Difficulties with chewing and swallowing
- Taking a very long time to complete meals
- Overall greater effort needed to eat or drink

Shortness of Breath

Patients may experience shortness of breath if the muscles of the chest cavity are affected by PD. Rigidity of the chest muscles may occur in general or during "off" periods as the dose of medicine is waning or during "on" periods when dyskinesia (involuntary movements) develops resulting in insufficient expansion of the chest muscles.

Visual Disturbances

Visual disturbances may appear in the absence of eye disease or poor visual acuity. The patient may have problems distinguishing objects that are the same color in anything less than very bright light. The reduction of visual contrast can interfere not only with daily activities but also in possibly not seeing objects on the floor, causing the patient to trip and/or fall.

As Parkinson's disease progresses, the severity of motor and non-motor symptoms increases as well. For example, falling becomes a greater problem as balance and walking deteriorate; or nighttime problems may increase due to frequent urination, muscular pain, and difficulty moving in bed, which compounds the issue of fatigue. Each stage requires careful evaluation in order to optimize the quality of life for the patient. In older people, quality of life may be even more affected because of impairments that occur with the "normal" aging process and compound the symptoms of Parkinson's disease. In advanced stages, the need for allied supportive health professionals increases since more severe disabilities require more physical and emotional support.

Diagnostic Testing for Parkinson's Disease

Currently, there are no blood tests or imaging scans to accurately diagnose Parkinson's disease (PD). The clinical diagnosis of PD is determined by evaluation of the patient's symptoms and clinical presentation. It is very important that the physician examining the patient (usually a neurologist) have the skill and experience needed for diagnosing movement disorders since Parkinson's disease is misdiagnosed in 25-35% of cases. The incidence of misdiagnosis declines sharply when the patient is evaluated by a doctor who specializes in Parkinson's disease and other movement disorders.

The diagnosis of PD is difficult and in some cases may be a diagnosis based on the exclusion of other medical conditions. Typically, the neurological exam is the most revealing aspect of the overall diagnosis but if it remains unclear, the physician may request laboratory or imaging studies in order to rule out diseases that present with symptoms that are similar to those of PD. Following an in-depth physical examination, the doctor may proceed with:

- Neurological evaluation
- Laboratory evaluation
- Imaging Studies

Neurological Evaluation of Parkinson's Disease

The physician performs an in-depth neurological evaluation to determine which symptoms of TRAP are present (i.e., tremor at rest, rigidity, akinesia, and postural instability) and their severity. However, these symptoms do not always present themselves in a way that

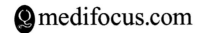

clearly points to Parkinson's disease.

Many physicians use a test called the Unified Parkinson's Disease Rating Scale (UPDRS), which is a very sensitive indicator of signs of early Parkinson's disease in particular and of the presence Parkinson's disease symptoms in general. The sections of the UPDRS are described above.

- The first part consists of information collected from the patient and family members regarding the difficulty of performing routine activities of daily living at home, (e.g., dressing, bathing, showering, eating, walking).
- The last two parts of the test involve an intensive physical examination and neurological evaluation by the physician which focuses on the presence and severity of TRAP symptoms (e.g., getting out of a chair, walking with a normal stride, swinging the arms symmetrically).

Sometimes, to confirm a diagnosis of Parkinson's disease, the physician may prescribe antiparkinson dopamine-based medication to see if the patient shows improvement in walking, movements, or tremors. This information often rules out or establishes the diagnosis of Parkinson's disease, since most patients with classic PD respond to dopamine medication soon after it is initiated.

Laboratory Evaluation of Parkinson's Disease

Although there are no laboratory tests to establish the diagnosis of Parkinson's disease, many physicians order some of the following tests in order to rule out other underlying conditions:

- Complete blood count (CBC)
- Liver function test
- Thyroid function test
- Drug/Toxicology screen
- Serum ceruloplasmin (a copper-carrying protein) and 24-hour urine copper excretion
- Liver biopsy

Imaging Studies for Parkinson's Disease

If the diagnosis is still not clear after physical and neurological evaluation, the physician may order neuroimaging tests, including:

- *Positron Emission Tomography* (PET Scan) in which a radioactive tracer such as 18-fluorodopa is injected intravenously while a scanner measures the uptake of the tracer in the substantia nigra portion of the midbrain and thus determines the number of dopamine cells present.

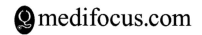

- *Single Photon Emission Computed Tomography* (SPECT) which is similar to a PET scan but uses a different radioactive tracer and measures the uptake of the material in the brain differently.

These scans are rarely ordered since they are very expensive and not always covered by insurance.

Differential Diagnosis of Parkinson's Disease

Several other conditions can mimic the neurologic symptoms of Parkinson's disease and must be excluded before the diagnosis is established. It is important to differentiate between true idiopathic (unknown cause) Parkinson's disease and parkinsonian symptoms that develop secondary to some underlying condition or medication.

The three most common categories of conditions that may be mistaken for Parkinson's disease include *medication-induced parkinsonism*, *Parkinson-plus syndrome*, and *essential tremor*.

- Medication-induced parkinsonism - Certain medications may either cause parkinsonian symptoms or exacerbate the severity of symptoms in the individual diagnosed with Parkinson's disease. It is important to determine whether symptoms are related to medications, in which case discontinuing the medications can result in cessation of symptoms over time, or to actual Parkinson's disease. The most common medications that can induce parkinsonian symptoms include:

    - *antipsychotics* - Examples include haloperidol, thioridazine (Mellaril), risperidone (Risperdal), lithium (Eskalith), chlorpromazine (Thorazine), and olanzapine (Zyprexa). Parkinsonian side-effects of these medications can last 1-2 years after stopping the medications.
    - *antiemetics* - These drugs are used to treat nausea and vomiting. Examples include prochlorperazine (Compazine) and metoclopramide (Reglan).
    - *antihypertensives* - These drugs are used to treat high blood pressure. Examples include methyldopa (Aldomet) and reserpine (Harmonyl).
    - *antianginals* - Heart medications used to treat angina or chest pain such as dilitiazem (Cardizem).
    - *antineoplastics* - These drugs are used to treat various types of cancers.

- Parkinson-Plus syndromes - This is a group of disorders which presents with parkinsonism in association with other distinct clinical features, such as autonomic disturbances (Shy-Drager syndrome) or ataxia (multi-system atrophy). These syndromes show poor or short-lived therapeutic response to Parkinson's disease medications and include symptoms or patterns of symptoms that do not appear in Parkinson's disease such as:

- signs of dementia early after onset of symptoms
- incidences of falling soon after onset of symptoms
- feet set wide apart while walking
- abnormal eye movements
- symmetric (bilateral) signs of parkinsonism
- severe disability within five years of onset of symptoms

- Essential tremor - tremors that are similar to those of PD but are identified based on the following characteristics:

  - typically bilateral
  - often accompanied by head tremor or tremulous voice
  - handwriting is typically large and tremulous
  - signs of bradykinesia and rigidity are absent

Other conditions which should be ruled out when a patient presents with Parkinson-like symptoms include:

- Multi-infarct disease (multiple small strokes), also called *arteriosclerotic* or *vascular parkinsonism*.
- Other degenerative brain diseases such as Alzheimer's disease (destroys memory and cognition) and Huntington's disease (causes uncontrolled movements and cognitive loss). Parkinsonian features occur in many patients with Alzheimer's disease and other dementias.
- Dementia with Lewy bodies.
- Normal Pressure Hydrocephalus which is an excessive accumulation of cerebrospinal fluid in the cerebral ventricles of the brain.
- Brain tumors.
- Exposure to toxins such as manganese dust, carbon disulfide and carbon monoxide
- Abuse of drugs containing MPTP(1-methyl-4-phenyl-1,2,3,6-tetrahydropyridine), often found in heroin, which was found to cause a permanent form of Parkinson's. This finding in the 1980's actually heralded an important breakthrough in Parkinson's disease research as scientists could induce a simulated Parkinson's disease in animals for further study.
- Shuffling gait disorders which can be caused by many other conditions and are often misdiagnosed as Parkinson's disease.

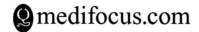

- Wilson's disease which causes the body to retain copper

Clinical features of PD that distinguish it from these conditions include:

- Asymmetry of motor symptoms
- Tremors at rest
- Good to excellent response to levodopa-based medications

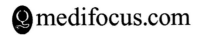

Treatment Options for Parkinson's Disease

Goals of Treatment for Parkinson's Disease

Treatment for Parkinson's disease is highly individualized. The goal of therapy is to reduce symptoms and improve quality of life while minimizing side effects of medications. The decision to treat early Parkinson's disease with pharmacological agents often depends on the particular needs of the person and careful weighing of possible benefits, cost, and adverse outcomes. Doctors try to use the lowest dose of any medications to achieve satisfactory improvement of function.

At the present time, there is no universally accepted standard of care - either in terms of how to treat early symptoms, the optimum time to start treatment, or which medications should be given for initial treatment of Parkinson's disease. It is also difficult to set a standard of care because the response of each individual to medication can be so varied.

There is currently no cure for Parkinson's disease. With the initial diagnosis of Parkinson's disease, the patient and doctor must determine the level of discomfort or inconvenience of the symptoms in daily life and, based on these findings, establish the initial decisions for therapy. There are three categories of treatments for Parkinson's disease to minimize symptoms and maximize function and quality of life, namely:

- Lifestyle modifications
- Pharmacological therapy
- Surgical therapy

Lifestyle Modifications for Parkinson's Disease

There is general agreement that the first line of therapy for mild symptoms in early Parkinson's disease is lifestyle modifications. This approach alone, however, is usually not sufficient once the symptoms begin to interfere with activities of daily living. Lifestyle modifications effective for early Parkinson's disease (PD) include:

- Education
- Exercise
- Nutrition

Education
The patient and family are encouraged to learn as much about Parkinson's disease as possible including issues related to:

- Knowledge about the disease
- Signs of symptom progression and treatment options
- Variations in the rate of progression of disease among patients
- Support services available in the community
- Emotional needs of patients and caregivers
- Coping strategies for disabilities
- Help available for home care
- Respite care options

Exercise

This is considered the most important adjunct therapy for all stages of Parkinson's disease. Though it does not affect the progression of Parkinson's disease, it has a very positive effect on mobility and mood of the patient. It also helps the patient retain as much function as possible in each stage of disease. Exercise should be carried out under the guidance of a physical therapist who can respond to the changing needs of the Parkinson's disease patient as the disease progresses.

The types of exercises that are most important are:

- Aerobics
- Strengthening exercises
- Stretching exercises
- Balance training

Activities such as walking, swimming, or gardening are beneficial and some researchers believe that weight-bearing exercises (such as walking) are especially helpful. Since energy levels fluctuate, it is important for Parkinson's disease patients to pace themselves when performing these activities. Balance training is crucial because postural instability increases with duration and severity of PD and raises the risk of falling and subsequent injury.

Exercise needs to be done consistently. Physical therapists suggest exercising for 20 minutes, three times a week depending upon flexibility and fatigue level. Emphasis of exercise should be strengthening and stretching extensor muscles to counteract the flexors, which become rigid with disease progression. As Parkinson's symptoms progress, physical therapy plays an increasingly important role for maintaining limb mobility and range of movement.

Nutrition

It is important for the Parkinson's disease patient to eat a healthy diet with adequate fruits, vegetables, and whole grains to optimize health at every stage. In addition, vigilance regarding regular mealtimes and eating habits is necessary since PD patients are at

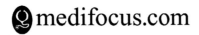

increased risk for weight loss and loss of muscle mass. Good dietary habits are also helpful in preventing or alleviating some gastrointestinal symptoms of PD such as constipation.

Protein acts as a competitor with dopamine when it comes to being metabolized by the body. As a result, doctors recommend that patients not eat any protein for 30-45 minutes before and after taking levodopa-related medications.

The position of the American Academy of Neurology is that there is no therapeutic or neuroprotective benefit to the nutritional supplement tocopherol (Vitamin E). However, there is ongoing investigation of the neuroprotective properties of Coenzyme Q10, a dietary supplement that is not regulated or approved by the U.S. Food and Drug Administration (FDA).

To read more about the study on Vitamin E and Parkinson's disease, please click on the following link: http://www.ncbi.nlm.nih.gov/pubmed/16622156

To read more about the position of the National Institute of Neurological Disorders and Stroke on Coenzyme Q10 and Parkinson's disease, please click on the following link: http://www.ninds.nih.gov/newsandevents/newsarticles/pressreleaseparkinsons coenzymeq10101402.htm

To read more about neuroprotection and nutritional supplements and Parkinson's Disease, please click on the following links: http://www.ncbi.nlm.nih.gov/pubmed/18394564 and http://www.ncbi.nlm.nih.gov/pubmed/16639735

Drug Therapy for Parkinson's Disease

Since the underlying disease process of Parkinson's disease involves the death of dopamine-producing cells and the subsequent reduction of dopamine available in the brain, one of the objectives of treatment is to increase the amount of dopamine by using agents that either:

- Increase dopamine levels in the brain
- Stimulate dopamine receptors in the brain
- Slow the metabolism and breakdown of dopamine in the brain and reduce the fluctuations of dopamine in the blood

To meet these objectives, there are several categories of medication used to treat Parkinson's disease, namely:

- Dopaminergic agents - increase levels of production of dopamine

  - *levodopa* which is converted by the brain into dopamine.

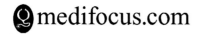

- *dopamine agonists* which stimulate the dopamine receptors in the brain by mimicking the effects of dopamine and cause the neurons to behave as if there was enough dopamine present to function smoothly.
  - *Neupro transdermal patch*

- *MAO-B inhibitors* that slow the breakdown of dopamine in the brain.

- *COMT inhibitors* that block COMT, an enzyme that metabolizes levodopa.
- *Anticholinergics* that block specific nerve impulses (cholinergic) that help control the muscles of the arms, legs, and body.
- *Cholinesterase inhibitors* that increase the levels of acetylcholine in the brain.
- *Amantadine* (Symmetrel) which is an *antiviral drug* that is believed to release dopamine from nerve endings in the brain making it more available to activate dopaminergic receptors.

Anticholinergics and amantadine alone are only mildly to moderately effective and are used only in combination with other medications.

Dopaminergic Medication
Levodopa

Until recently, levodopa was considered the "golden drug" for initial symptomatic treatment of Parkinson's disease. It became available in the 1960's and represented the first dramatic breakthrough in the treatment of Parkinson's disease. It is a highly effective drug and has been shown to extend life expectancy in Parkinson's disease patients. Before levodopa was introduced, the only agent that could relieve Parkinson's disease symptoms was anticholinergic drugs for the relief of rigidity and resting tremor. Levodopa is most effective for bradykinesia (slowness of movement) and rigidity. It is less effective for resting tremor.

Levodopa brought about a revolution in Parkinson's disease treatment by reversing the neurochemical abnormality responsible for the symptoms and making dopamine available for the brain. Dopamine itself cannot cross the blood/brain barrier (a tight "net" of blood vessels that protects the brain by preventing many agents from crossing into the brain). Levodopa was the first drug that was formulated in such a way that some dopamine was able to reach the brain.

Sinemet (levodopa combined with carbidopa) is the standard formulation of levodopa for Parkinson's disease patients today. This was a significant modification of levodopa because while carbidopa does not cross the blood brain barrier, it inhibits levodopa from being metabolized into dopamine in the digestive system (outside the central nervous system) and leaves a greater concentration of levodopa available to reach the brain with each dose.

Thus, Sinemet reduces the amount of levodopa necessary to achieve desired motor control. Sinemet also minimizes some of the short term side effects of pure levodopa, including nausea and vomiting.

When a Parkinson's disease patient begins treatment with levodopa, there is a dramatic improvement of symptoms. However, as time progresses, the patient begins to find that the Parkinson's symptoms recur and the dose to achieve comfort may need to be raised. Combining levodopa, carbidopa and entacapone (a COMT inhibitor) in a drug called *Stalevo*, has been found to prolong the action of levodopa, thereby providing relief with lower doses of levodopa.

There is a slow, sustained-release formulation of Sinemet available which reduces the uncomfortable side effects. The controlled-release Sinemet is only moderately effective and does not significantly reduce motor complications in most patients. Some doctors prescribe the slow release Sinemet to be taken as the last dose before the patient goes to bed.

Levodopa is considered to be so effective for Parkinson's disease that only approximately 10% of patients with Parkinson's disease do not respond. Indeed, some physicians are of the opinion that if a patient with parkinsonian symptoms does not respond to levodopa, other causes for the symptoms should be investigated.

Over time, patients taking increasingly large doses of levodopa find that not only is the effectiveness reduced but major side-effects become evident. This typically takes place in about 50% of the patients after approximately five years. Some of these events occur because levodopa has a short half-life (the time it takes for half the dose of the drug to be eliminated from the body) of approximately 1.5 hours so the effect of the drug wears off quickly and symptoms reappear.

Side-effects of levodopa can have a profound effect on the quality of life of the patient and include:

- Dyskinesia - involuntary movements (e.g., twitching, nodding, or jerking). The movements can be mild or severe, slow or rapid. The only way to control them is to cut back on the amount of levodopa, but a return of Parkinson symptoms such as rigidity quickly recurs. At this point, other medications are utilized. This is the most problematic side effect of levodopa and has a significant negative impact on quality of life.

- "Wearing-off" effect - this is the deterioration of symptoms that occurs when levodopa wears off. It may be an indication that the patient must take the drug more frequently. Often, the patient experiences symptoms of dystonia (involuntary muscle

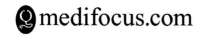

spasms which can cause abnormal movements).

- "On-off" effect - also called the "yo-yo" phenomenon, which is due to the fluctuation of dopamine levels in the blood. The patient experiences sudden, unpredictable changes in the ability to move. They may go from carrying out a motor activity normally ("on") to suddenly freezing or becoming totally rigid with parkinsonian symptoms ("off"). This can happen several times a day. The "on-off" effect usually indicates either that the patient's response to levodopa is changing or that the disease is progressing.

- Parkinsonian symptoms are more intense before the patient takes the first dose of levodopa in the morning.

- Hallucinations

- Restlessness

- Orthostatic hypotension (drop in blood pressure when standing after sitting)

When levodopa is introduced to patients with Young-Onset Parkinson's Disease, the response to the first dose is dramatic but they are likely to develop associated side effects, primarily dyskinesia, after a few months of taking the drug. Those with adult onset of Parkinson's disease usually manifest the same side effects after an average of three to five years.

On August 20, 2010 the FDA notified healthcare professionals that it is evaluating clinical trial data that suggest patients taking Stalevo (a combination of carbidopa/levodopa plus entacapone) may be at increased risk for cardiovascular events such as heart attack, stroke, and cardiovascular death compared to patients taking carbidopa/levodopa without entacapone (sold as the combination product, Sinemet).

Both Stalevo and Sinemet have been shown to be effective treatments for reducing the symptoms of Parkinson's disease.

The FDA's decision to review the data of clinical trials was based on findings from the Stalevo Reduction in Dyskinesia - Parkinson's Disease or STRIDE-PD trial, which reported an imbalance in the number of heart attacks in patients treated with Stalevo compared to those receiving only carbidopa/levodopa. Although heart attack, cardiac irregularities, high blood pressure, and heart palpitations have been reported with levodopa, previous clinical trials with Stalevo did not show an in imbalance in heart attacks, stroke, and cardiovascular deaths.

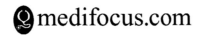

At this time, the FDA's review of potential cardiovascular risks associated with Stalevo is still ongoing. In the meantime, until its review of the clinical trial data has been completed, the FDA issued the following recommendations for healthcare professionals and patients:

- Healthcare professionals should regularly evaluate the cardiovascular status of patients who are taking Stalevo, particularly if they have a history of cardiovascular disease.

- Patients should not stop taking Stalevo unless told so by their healthcare professional.

- The FDA will update the public about its findings when this review of Stalevo has been completed.

Dopamine Agonists

Dopamine agonists mimic the effects of dopamine in the brain and cause neurons to react as if there were enough dopamine present to carry out their function. This class of medications is used either as a monotherapy (single drug) or in combination with levodopa. If used initially as a single therapy, after a certain amount of time, levodopa is added because the relief that the dopamine agonists provide is not sufficient to reduce the symptoms and improve the quality of life as the disease progresses. If levodopa is used as the initial therapy, the dopamine agonists are added in order to prolong the duration that dopamine is active in the brain and thus reduce the "wearing off" effect and dyskinesia.

Dopamine agonists used to treat the symptoms of PD include:

- Ropinirole (Requip) - used alone or with other medications
- Pramipexole (Mirapex) - used alone or with other medications
- Bromocriptine (Parlodel) - used alone or with other medications and works by stimulating the nerves that control movement.
- Apomorphine (Apokyn) - used to treat "off" episodes (such as difficulty moving, walking, and speaking) that occur as a dose wears off. Apomorphine will not prevent "off" episodes, but will help improve symptoms when an "off" episode has already begun.
- Pergolide (Permax) - In March 2007, the FDA notified healthcare professionals and patients that pergolide has been withdrawn from the market because it has been linked to serious damage to heart valves.
- Lisuride (Dopergin) - not available in the U.S.
- Cabergoline (Cabaser) - not available in the U.S.

- Neupro transdermal patch (Rotigotine) - presently not approved by the U.S. Food & Drug Administration.

Dopamine agonists are not as effective as levodopa particularly in alleviating rigidity and bradykinesia. However some doctors feel that since dopamine agonists do have some beneficial effect on parkinsonian symptoms, and the side effects are not as severe as those of levodopa, it is worthwhile to initially prescribe a dopamine agonist for mild symptoms and then add levodopa later as needed. Some studies indicate that dopamine agonists as monotherapy can reduce symptoms for up to three years and reduce the risk of developing side effects (dyskinesia and motor fluctuations) for up to four or five years. Another advantage of dopamine agonists is that they have a longer half-life than levodopa. Their use does not induce the "wearing off" effect or dyskinesia and may actually moderate these effects when combined with levodopa.

In studies comparing quality of life in PD patients that took levodopa or dopamine agonists over a period of four years, the resulting quality of life scores were comparable, though there were fewer dyskinesias reported for those patients taking the dopamine agonists (pramipexole or ropinirole). More long-term data is necessary before decisions can be made to reduce reliance on levodopa.

One of the major decisions that needs to be made by the patient and the doctor is whether using dopamine agonists to delay dyskinesia and possibly delay disease progression is worth the poorer control of motor symptoms which are so effectively reduced by levodopa. In addition, dopamine agonists are associated with more side effects when used as a monotherapy than when combined with levodopa.

An additional issue that doctors should consider before prescribing dopamine agonists is the burden of cost on the patient, since dopamine agonists are significantly more expensive than levodopa.

Dopamine agonists do have some significant side-effects, some of which are cognitive in nature and can significantly interfere with daily living. These include:

- Paranoia
- Hallucinations
- Confusion
- Nightmares
- Nausea
- Vomiting

Some patients develop dyskinesia as well but these are usually not as severe as those seen following levodopa.

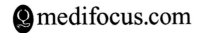
Because of the nature of these complications, dopamine agonists are not given to patients who already suffer from any type of cognitive impairment. Recent data has shown a possible link between ergot-based dopamine agonists, such as bromocriptine (Parlodel) and pergolide (Permax), and dysfunction of cardiac valves. As a result, non-ergot based dopamine agonists such as ropinirole (Requip) and pramipexole (Mirapex) should be tried first.

In general, the data so far suggests that dopamine agonists are a significant addition to the arsenal of drugs that are effective in reducing symptoms of Parkinson's disease as well as moderating the side effects associated with levodopa. However, because response to the drugs is so variable, each doctor must evaluate carefully with the patient the choice of drugs as well as the timetable for adding or combining new drugs.

In 2007, *rotigotine* was formulated as a *transdermal delivery system* called the *Neupro patch* for the treatment of patients with early Parkinson's disease. The patch is applied once a day to the skin and continuously releases the drug through the skin for a 24-hour period.

In March 2008, the manufacturer of Neupro (Schwarz Pharma) informed healthcare professionals and patients of the recall of Neupro because of the formation of rotigotine crystals in the patches. When the rotigotine crystallizes, less drug is available to be absorbed through the skin and, therefore, the efficacy of the product may vary. Neupro was reformulated and in June 2009, received approval for use for treatment of mild symptoms of PD in Europe. Neupro is currently under review by the FDA but has not received approval to date.

Monoamine Oxidase Type-B (MAO-B) Inhibitors

There are two MAO-B inhibitors used in the treatment of Parkinson's disease, *selegiline* (Eldepryl) and *rasagiline* (Azilect). Dopamine is one of the brain chemicals known as *monoamines* which are broken down by a protein known as *oxidase*. MAO-B inhibitors limit the action of oxidase and prevent the breakdown of dopamine in the brain resulting in an enhanced and prolonged effect of levodopa. There has also been considerable debate as to whether the MAO-B inhibitors used for Parkinson's disease are neuroprotective and possibly delay the progression of Parkinson's disease.

Selegiline

The most widely used MAO-B inhibitor is selegiline (Eldepryl, Deprenyl). Selegiline is used as an adjunct to levodopa since it increases the half-life of dopamine in the brain. There has been considerable debate as to whether selegiline is neuroprotective and possibly delays the progression of Parkinson's disease.

When given to patients in the early-stage PD as a monotherapy, some studies suggest that selegiline delays the need for Sinemet possibly by as long as nine months. Other studies have shown that there is no support for giving selegiline as an initial monotherapy. When given later in disease progression, selegiline boosts the effect of levodopa and improves the problem of fluctuations of motor response in about one half to two thirds of patients. The drug is easily tolerated. In general, selegiline is considered to be only moderately effective resulting in its being prescribed more as an adjunct medication rather than as a monotherapy.

Side effects of selegiline include:

- Nausea
- Orthostatic hypotension (low blood pressure when changing from a sitting to standing position)
- Insomnia
- Confusion
- Abdominal pain

Rasagiline

On May 17, 2006, the U.S. Food and Drug Administration (FDA) approved a newer MAO-B inhibitor called rasagiline (Azilect) for the treatment of Parkinson's disease. This drug was approved for use as an initial single drug therapy (monotherapy) for patients with early Parkinson's disease and in combination with levodopa in patients with more advanced Parkinson's disease. Various studies have indicated that when used in levodopa-treated patients, rasagiline is effective for:

- Reducing motor fluctuations
- Reducing average daily "off" time
- Improving UPDRS scores for activities of daily living

When rasagiline was studied as a monotherapy for treatment of early PD, total UPDRS scores improved by 30% or more. Studies are ongoing regarding the possibility of rasagiline slowing the rate of progression of Parkinson's disease. To read the results of a recent study in the *New England Journal of Medicine* of September 2009 that evaluated a delayed start of rasagiline in untreated PD patients by comparing a group who received rasagiline for 72 weeks with a group that received a placebo for 36 weeks and then rasagiline for 36 weeks, please click on the following link:
http://www.ncbi.nlm.nih.gov/pubmed/19776408

Rasagiline is well tolerated and is not associated with side effects.

A study published in 2005 in the *British Journal of Cancer* (Volume 92, Issue 1; pp. 201-205) reported that Parkinson's disease patients may be at increased risk for developing

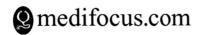

a type of skin cancer known as *malignant melanoma*. This type of skin cancer was also diagnosed in a small number of patients treated with rasagiline. Although there is no clear evidence that rasagiline is associated with an increased risk of melanoma, current recommendations suggest that patients receiving treatment with rasagiline should undergo periodic check-ups from a dermatologist to monitor any signs of development of melanoma and other types of skin cancer.

While taking MAO-B inhibitors, caution must be taken regarding adverse drug interactions with other medications, including many nonprescription cold medications that contain pseudoephedrine, (a decongestant) and dextromethorphan (a cough suppressant).

Catechol-O-Methyltransferase (COMT) Inhibitors

- Tolcapone (Tasmar)
- Entacapone (Comtan)

COMT inhibitors prolong the effect of levodopa by blocking the enzyme known as catechol-O-methyltransferase (COMT) that breaks down dopamine in the liver and other organs. As a result, many of the adverse effects of levodopa which result because of sudden drops or fluctuations in the levels of levodopa are reduced. This reduces the "off" duration which is seen in motor complications of levodopa. COMT inhibitors also decrease the "wearing off" effect.

Tolcapone

Tolcapone (Tasmar) is a very potent drug which easily crosses the blood/brain barrier and is used as an adjunct to levodopa. Because it increases the half-life of levodopa, the patient can reduce levodopa intake by 25-30%.

The major side effect of tolcapone is liver toxicity leading to liver failure. Because of this, tolcapone is given only to Parkinson's disease patients who are not responding to other medications. Once a patient begins taking tolcapone, they require very close monitoring of liver function. The FDA suggests that patients be monitored every two weeks for the first year; then every four weeks for the following six months; and every eight weeks, thereafter. The FDA also suggests that if a patient does not exhibit substantial improvement within the first three weeks of taking the first dose, the drug should be withdrawn.

Other adverse effects of tolcapone may include:

- Dyskinesia
- Nausea
- Sleep disorder
- Muscle cramps

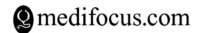
Entacapone

Entacapone (Comtan) is similar in composition to tolcapone but does not cross the blood/brain barrier. It is used as an adjunct to levodopa and is effective in reducing the "wearing-off" effect. Because of the lower risk of complications involved with this drug, it is the COMT inhibitor usually prescribed.

The main adverse effects associated with entacapone include:

- Urine discoloration
- Nausea
- Dyskinesia

Anticholinergic Agents

Examples of anticholinergic medications that may be used to better control tremor in patients with Parkinson's disease include:

- Trihexyphenidyl (Artane)
- Benztropine (Cogentin)
- Biperiden (Akineton)
- Diphenhydramine (Benadryl)
- Procyclidine (Kemadrin)

Anticholinergic agents do not act directly on dopamine as do the other drugs previously mentioned. Rather, they decrease the effect of acetylcholine which counteracts the benefits of dopamine in the brain. They are most effective for the control of tremor. Even so, they are only moderately beneficial.

Anticholinergics were the drug of choice for Parkinson's disease before the discovery of levodopa. Since only about half the people who take anticholinergics respond, and even then only for a brief time, they are not used often. Also, since tremors are often not such a disabling aspect of Parkinson's symptoms there is less need to add this medication to control them.

Adverse effects associated with anticholinergic medications include:

- Dry mouth
- Nausea
- Urine retention
- Constipation
- Memory loss
- Confusion

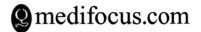 **medifocus.com**

- Hallucinations

Because of the side effects, anticholinergics are rarely prescribed people over 70 years of age or for any patient already experiencing mental impairment. In some circumstances, doctors find that older people who cannot tolerate anticholinergics may tolerate antihistamines (e.g., Benadryl) and antidepressants (e.g., Elavil) that have similar effects on Parkinson's symptoms. In general, anticholinergic drugs are not widely used in treatment of Parkinson's disease because of their minimal efficacy and the side effects associated with them.

Cholinesterase Inhibitors

Cholinesterase inhibitors are a class of drugs that help to increase both the levels and duration of action of the neurotransmitter *acetylcholine* in the brain. Acetylcholine plays an important role in learning and memory and low levels of acetylcholine in the brain are associated with dementia and Alzheimer's disease. Cholinesterase inhibitors, which inhibit the breakdown of acetylcholine by an enzyme called *cholinesterase*, are used to treat cognitive impairment and dementia that are relatively common features of Parkinson's disease.

Risk factors for Parkinson's disease-related dementia include:

- Advanced age (age 70 or older)
- A score of 25 or higher on the Parkinson's Disase Rating Scale
- Adverse psychological response to treatment with levodopa (depression, agitation, or psychotic behavior)
- Exposure to severe psychological stress
- History of cardiovascular disease

Examples of cholinesterase inhibitors that may be used to treat Parkinson's disease-related dementia include:

- Donepezil (Aricept)
- Galantamine (Reminyl)
- Rivastigmine (Exelon) - available either as an oral formulation (capsules) or as a transdermal patch designed for adminstration through the skin.

Adverse effects of cholinesterase inhibitors may include:

- Anorexia
- Nausea
- Vomiting
- Diarrhea

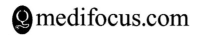

• Insomnia

Antiviral Drugs

The most commonly used antiviral drug is *amantadine* (Symmetrel) which reduces symptoms of Parkinson's disease by blocking the reuptake of dopamine resulting in an increase in the availability of dopamine in the brain. After several months, the effectiveness wears off in approximately one-third to one-half of the patients. Amantadine is most useful to treat levodopa-induced dyskinesia. Amantadine is considered as only moderately effective resulting in its being prescribed more as an add-on medication rather than as a monotherapy.

Side effects of amantadine include significant cognitive impairment (e.g., hallucinations) and for this reason, it is usually not given to older people or to people who already experience cognitive symptoms. Other side effects include:

• Blurred vision
• Depression
• Edema
• Confusion

Other Medications for Parkinson's Disease

There are several other medications that have not been approved by the FDA for treatment of Parkinson's disease symptoms but may be used to help control various symptoms. For example, *botulinum toxin* injections may be administered to reduce saliva production and drooling. *Collagen* injections may help voice and speech disorders by augmenting the vocal fold.

Neuroprotective Therapy for Parkinson's Disease

The goal of neuroprotective therapy is to prevent or delay the progression of PD by protecting the neurons from damage caused by biochemical changes that result in the loss of dopamine. The rationale for seeking neuroprotective agents is that typically at the time of diagnosis with PD, approximately 40% of the dopamine-producing cells are still functioning and it is important to protect them from injury. There are many studies being conducted to evaluate various potentially neuroprotective agents including:

• Coenzyme Q10 (ubidecarenone)- an antioxidant
• Certain dopamine agonists - so far the indications are that the only dopamine agonist that might do so is pramipexole and possibly ropinirole. However, the current evidence is inconclusive and no definitive conclusions have been reached.
• MAO-B inhibitors (selegiline, rasagiline)

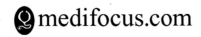

A Practice Parameter published by the American Academy of Neurology (AAN) in 2006 indicated that no treatment to date has been shown to be neuroprotective. To read more about the conclusions of the AAN regarding neuroprotective agents and Parkinson's disease, please click on the following link:

http://www.ncbi.nlm.nih.gov/pubmed/16606908

Neuroleptic Malignant Syndrome

Neuroleptic Malignant Syndrome (NMS) is a rare complication of Parkinson's disease and is usually triggered by a reduction or discontinuation of antiparkinsonian drugs, especially, but not exclusively, levodopa. Additional triggers for NMS are infection and dehydration. Symptoms include high fever, increased rigidity and exacerbation of Parkinson's disease symptoms, disturbances of consciousness, disturbances of the autonomic system (including blood pressure), and elevated creatine kinase levels in the blood.

It is critical for Neuroleptic Malignant Syndrome to be treated immediately as it can lead to pneumonia or renal failure. Treatment usually includes infusion of intravenous fluids, cooling to bring down fever, increasing or reintroducing antiparkinsonian medication, as well as administration of other drugs such as bromocriptine (Parlodel) and dantrolene (Dantrium). There is ongoing research into the efficacy of other medications in treating NMS.

Surgical Therapy for Parkinson's Disease

Surgical intervention was relatively common for the treatment of Parkinson's disease before the introduction of levodopa. It then fell out of practice but is now being re-evaluated as new surgical techniques become available.

Surgery may be recommended as a treatment for:

- Young-Onset Parkinson's Disease patients for whom drugs do not adequately control the symptoms and who have no evidence of cognitive impairment or other medical problems.
- Patients of any age with advanced stage Parkinson's disease who are no longer responsive to medication and who suffer from disabling tremors or associated Parkinson's disease "off-period" symptoms such as motor fluctuations or dyskinesia.
- Parkinson's disease patients of any age who have a significantly impaired quality of life due to PD-related motor symptoms.

Surgery is not curative and is intended only to relieve symptoms of Parkinson's disease. Since the symptoms which may warrant surgery are associated with advanced Parkinson's

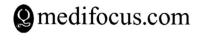

disease, surgical intervention is not considered as an option for early Parkinson's disease.

Currently, there are two types of surgical procedures that may be considered for Parkinson's disease patients:

- Ablation (destruction of tissue)
- Stimulation

Both procedures target highly specific areas of the brain but whereas ablation involves the destruction of the tissue, stimulation provides electrical stimulation to the tissue. Ablation and stimulation are performed via needle-guided stereotactic brain surgery. Before surgery, the patient undergoes several imaging studies in order to pinpoint the target area and other structures that lie in close proximity. During the procedure, the patient is not fully anesthetized since they need to communicate with the surgeon's questions about the sensations they are feeling at particular moments. Their responses help the surgeon determine if the electrode is correctly placed since incorrect placement results in "incorrect" sensations such as seeing flashing lights. There is no pain involved in the actual placement of the electrode as there are no pain sensors in the brain itself. However, local anesthesia is given during the preparatory stages of accessing the brain.

There are three targeted areas of the brain in which these surgical procedures are performed:

- Globus pallidus internus (GPi)
- Thalamus
- Subthalamic nucleus (STN)

If your doctor recommends surgery for Parkinson's disease, it is important to confirm coverage for these procedures with your health insurance carrier before undergoing the procedure.

Ablation

This type of surgery involves the destruction of targeted brain tissue via delivery of radiofrequency energy. Until the 1990s, this was the most common type of surgery for PD, but is presently not as frequently used due to more effective surgical procedures and the high risk of complications. Two types of ablation surgery performed for symptoms of PD are *pallidotomy* and *thalamotomy*.

Pallidotomy

Pallidotomy is performed to treat:

- Peak-dose dyskinesia (uncontrolled movements that occur when levodopa is at its highest concentration in the blood)
- "Wearing-off" dystonia (muscle spasms at the lowest concentration of levodopa as the medication wears off)
- Bradykinesia and tremor - pallidotomy is not as effective for these symptoms

Pallidotomy involves the destruction of part of the globus pallidus internus (GPi) that controls movement. A wire probe is inserted into the GPi and the precise target location is identified by MRI. The probe is heated by radio waves to a temperature that destroys the tissue in the immediate area. Since the reduction and loss of dopamine cause overactivity in the GPi, destruction of part of the tissue restores the balance needed for controlled movement. Effects from the ablation are seen almost immediately.

Outcomes of pallidotomy are estimated to be 70-90% reduction of dyskinesia and 25-50% reduction of tremor, rigidity, bradykinesia, and gait disturbance. The dose of levodopa may be reduced following surgery.

Pallidotomy can be performed as a unilateral procedure where ablation is limited to one side of the brain or as a bilateral procedure. While bilateral pallidotomy is more effective for reducing dyskinesia, it is associated with a higher risk for complications involving cognition, speech, and swallowing and is rarely performed.

There are complications in approximately 10-20% of patients undergoing the pallidotomy procedure. Risks include the probe striking a blood vessel and causing a stroke, damaging adjacent areas, weakness, visual deficit, and confusion.

Thalamotomy

Thalamotomy is also a destructive (ablative) procedure during which a part of the thalamus (a structure below the GPi) is destroyed. It is effective for patients for whom tremor is the only disabling symptom. The ablation can be unilateral or bilateral but bilateral thalamotomy is associated with a higher risk of complications and is usually not performed. Thalalmotomy is rarely recommended for patients with PD.

Complications include hemorrhage, stroke, the probe damaging other major brain centers that are adjacent to the thalamus, worsening gait instability, and speech problems. Patients who exhibit these gait or speech problems prior to surgery are usually considered as candidates for the procedure.

Deep Brain Stimulation (DBS)

Deep brain stimulation is not a destructive procedure and does not ablate any tissue. Rather, an electrode is placed in the target location and is attached to a battery-operated programmable stimulator, about the size of a stopwatch, located in the chest wall that delivers continuous high-frequency electrical stimulation to the brain. Deep brain stimulation is a procedure based on evidence that loss of dopamine leads to abnormal activity in the GPi and STN. When electrical stimulation is delivered to one of those areas which are centers for movement control, the DBS effectively "paces" the cells and blocks or overrides any abnormal electrical activity.

Deep brain stimulation treatment is most effective for tremor, rigidity, stiffness, slowed movement (bradykinesia) and walking problems. Candidates for DBS include patients in whom control of symptoms with medication is inadequate. Patients who already underwent pallidotomy or thalamotomy are still considered eligible for DBS. Generally it has been noted that patients whose symptoms do not improve with levodopa are not responsive to DBS. Most patients will have to continue to take the medications they were taking for motor symptoms before the treatment but the doses may be reduced to reflect less intense symptoms.

Consideration of which brain structure is targeted for DBS is partially based on the following factors:

- *GPi* - stimulation of the GPi produces the greatest improvement for dyskinesia and more moderate improvement for tremor, rigidity, bradykinesia, and gait disturbances. Some patients can reduce the dosage of levodopa following this surgery. This surgery is also effective on patients suffering from dystonia. Bilateral deep brain stimulation of the GPi is well tolerated by many patients. Overall results of GPi stimulation are similar to those following pallidotomy.
- *Thalamus* - thalamic stimulation is most effective when the predominant symptom of PD is disabling tremor that it is stronger on one side of the body than the other. This procedure is reported to significantly reduce tremor in approximately two-thirds of the patients undergoing the surgery. Bilateral stimulation is possible but is associated with a higher risk of complications.
- *Subthalamic nucleus* - the STN has developed into a major target area for DBS and may in fact be the most effective location for alleviating symptoms of PD. Most motor features of Parkinson's disease, namely bradykinesia, tremor, and rigidity improve with DBS of the STN. Some patients can reduce the dosage of levodopa following surgery. This procedure is performed primarily on patient with advanced and disabling Parkinson's disease but ongoing studies are evaluating the efficacy for other PD patients as well. Advantages related to STN stimulation include:

    - motor symptoms are estimated to improve 40-60% during "off" periods
    - motor symptoms improve up to 10% during "on" periods
    - levodopa dose may be reduced up to 30% resulting in a reduction of dose-related dyskinesia

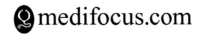

- bilateral DBS is superior to unilateral and is associated with only slightly increased risk of complications.

The procedure for implanting the device for deep brain stimulation begins with identifying the exact targeted area in the brain with either magnetic resonance imaging (MRI) or computed tomography (CT). The electrode (a thin insulated wire) is inserted into the brain through an opening in the skull and the tip is precisely placed in the targeted area. An insulated wire is passed under the skin of the head, neck, and shoulder and connected to the programmable stimulator which is usually implanted under the skin near the collarbone or over the abdomen.

Following surgery, the patient is taught how to control the stimulator to achieve maximum benefit of symptom control from DBS. Patients can also turn the stimulator off. It may take several weeks of adjusting the stimulator and medication before the full effect of DBS is achieved.

The U.S. Food & Drug Administration (FDA) approved DBS of the thalamus for the treatment of tremor in 1997, DBS of the STN in Parkinson's disease in 2002, and DBS of the GPi in 2003.

Possible complications include an electrode or wire leading to the battery becoming infected, or excessive bleeding that may occur if a blood vessel is penetrated. Stroke is also recognized as a risk factor of DBS. Hemorrhage or stroke occurs in approximately 1-3% of patients who undergo this surgical procedure.

The advantages of DBS include:

- Brain tissue is not destroyed and can be continuously treated or the electrical current can be turned off, if necessary.
- Better control of symptoms because placement of the electrode is more accurate.
- Less risk of stroke or hemorrhage.
- DBS can be reversed or easily adjusted for changing situations.
- A reduction of levodopa-associated dyskinesia.
- Motor fluctuations between "off" and "on" states are smoothed over.

The WeMove organization (www.wemove.org) notes that as DBS is being performed more frequently, rare but serious neuropsychiatric side effects are being observed, including the onset or worsening of depression and the depression-associated risk of suicide. A neuropsychological evaluation is recommended before performing DBS to identify patients with depression or those at increased risk for depression.

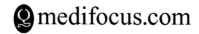

Experimental Procedures for Parkinson's Disease

There are several experimental procedures under active investigation for treatment of Parkinson's disease (PD) including:

- Fetal Cell Transplantation
- Gene Therapy

Fetal cell transplantation is an experimental procedure in which fetal brain cells from the substantia nigra that are rich in dopamine are implanted in the corpus striatum of the patient. The corpus striatum is involved in motor control and is easier and safer to locate than the substantia nigra which is smaller and deeper in the brain. This procedure is performed to restore dopamine levels in the brain and thus restore the patient to a less advanced stage of Parkinson's disease.

Several hundred fetal cell transplants have been performed with variable outcomes, ranging from no response to significant improvement. The agreed upon aspects of limited improvement include better motor control during "on" and "off" periods, an increase of "on" time, as well as a reduction of rigidity and bradykinesia. Results have been tracked from six months to several years. A reduction in the dose of dopamine may follow the surgery. Trials show that the greatest benefit of fetal cell transplantation is in younger Parkinson's disease patients. Because of the risk of rejection of the foreign fetal cells, the patient may be given immunosuppressive drugs indefinitely. The surgery is still considered experimental and the source of fetal cells is controversial for many doctors and patients.

Fetal cell transplantation is usually performed bilaterally, either in stages or simultaneously. Since not all fetal cells take effect with the procedure, an oversupply of fetal cells must be transplanted in hopes of reaching a critical mass of cells that will restore dopamine production. Benefits from the surgery are usually not seen for several months because the cells need time to propagate. In some patients, fetal tissue transplantation resulted in disabling dyskinesia. The risk of stroke or hemorrhage is approximately 1-3%.

To read more about fetal cell transplantation and PD, please click on the following link: http://www.ncbi.nlm.nih.gov/pubmed/19515281

Investigators are also studying the potential efficacy of *neural stem cells* for transplantation in PD. Stem cells are primitive cells that can grow into nerve cells that produce dopamine and can survive and reproduce. Research of stem cell transplantation for PD is in the very early stages of development.

A new approach at some clinical centers is the transplantation of retinal pigment cells from

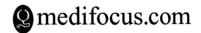
the tissue at the back of the eye into the striatum of patients with PD. Retinal cells are dopamine-producing cells. Results are based on small studies and look promising. To read more about this new procedure, please click on the following link:

http://www.ncbi.nlm.nih.gov/pubmed/18394567

Gene therapy involves the injection of genes (such as the glutamic acid decarboxylase or GAD gene) that control dopamine production into the neurons of the subthalamic nucleus. Results look promising and there are several clinical trials underway. Please click on the following link to read more about gene therapy and Parkinson's disease:
http://www.nlm.nih.gov/medlineplus/news/fullstory_90594.html

Guidelines for the Treatment of Parkinson's Disease

Medical management of Parkinson's disease consists of medication given either alone (monotherapy) or in combinations. There is considerable debate regarding which drugs to start first, when to combine drugs, and in what order. Regardless of which medication is chosen for treatment, the dose is initiated at the lowest level possible and then slowly increased until symptom relief is achieved and side effects are tolerable.

According to a Practice Parameter published by the American Academy of Neurology in 2002, the conclusions regarding initial treatment for Parkinson's disease include the following:

- First-line treatment of newly symptomatic Parkinson's disease patients should consist of either levodopa or dopamine agonists. Levodopa is more effective for symptomatic relief but carries greater risks for dyskinesia.
- Sustained release levodopa provides no advantage over the immediate release form of the drug.
- Selegiline, while of limited symptomatic benefit, has no neuroprotective properties.

In 2006, the Food and Drug Administration approved rasagiline as a monotherapy for treatment of early Parkinson's disease and as add-on therapy to levodopa for moderate and advanced stages.

The American Academy of Neurology published four additional Practice Parameters for the treatment of Parkinson's disease in *Neurology* in 2006 (vol 66(7): 968-975) in which the following conclusions were drawn:

Medical/Surgical Treatment for Levodopa-Induced Motor Fluctuations and Dyskinesia

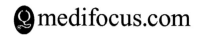

- To reduce "off" time dyskinesia:

  - Level A (highest) recommendation: entacapone and rasagiline
  - Level B: pergolide, pramipexole, ropinirole, and tolcapone
  - Level C: apomorphine, cabergoline, and selegeline

- Present evidence cannot recommend the superiority of one medication over another for reducing "off" time of drug dose.

- Sustained-release carbidopa/levodopa (Sinemet) and bromocriptine do not reduce "off" time.
- Amantadine (Symmetrel) may be considered to reduce dyskinesia (Level C)
- Deep brain stimulation (DBS) of the subthalamic nucleus (STN) may be considered (Level C) for:

  *improving motor function

  - reducing "off" time
  - reducing dyskinesia
  - reducing medication usage

- There is insufficient evidence to support or refute DBS in the globus pallidus internus (GPi) or thalamus for reducing "off" time, dyskinesia, or medication usage.

- Preoperative response to levodopa predicts better outcome for DBS of the STN.

More information about the AAN Guidelines for treating dyskinesia and motor fluctuations can be obtained by clicking on the following link:
http://www.ncbi.nlm.nih.gov/pubmed/16606909

Therapies that Slow Progression of PD or Affect Motor Function

- Levodopa does not accelerate disease progression.
- No treatment has been found to be neuroprotective.
- There is no evidence that any food additive or vitamin supplement improves motor function.
- Acupuncture may provide symptomatic benefit for motor and non-motor symptoms.
- Exercise may be helpful for improving motor function.
- Speech therapy may be helpful for improving speech volume.
- No manual therapy has been shown to be effective for improving motor symptoms.

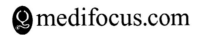

More information about the AAN Guidelines for neuroprotective agents and alternative medicine therapies that slow motor function decline in PD can be obtained by clicking on the following link: http://www.ncbi.nlm.nih.gov/pubmed/16606908

Therapies for Nonmotor Symptoms

- Amitriptyline can be recommended for depression.
- Clozapine (Level B) and quetiapine (Level C) can be used for treatment of psychosis but olanzapine should not be used.
- Donapezil or rivastigmine can be used for treatment of Parkinsons disease-related dementia. Rivastigmine (Exelon) is available either as an oral formulation (capsules) or as a patch designed for transdermal (via the skin) administration.

More information about the AAN Guidelines for therapies for nonmotor symptoms of PD can be obtained by clicking on the following link:
http://www.ncbi.nlm.nih.gov/pubmed/16606910

Treatment of Parkinson's patients is highly individualized and is based on many criteria. These include:

- Level of disability
- Stage of the disease
- Age of the patient
- Presence of comorbid conditions (e.g., dementia, hypertension)

Evaluation of these parameters helps determine when to introduce drug therapy and which classes of drugs to employ. Though there are no standard guidelines that are applicable for all patients, there are certain principles that seem to be widely accepted. These include:

- If the patient is below the age of 70, they will usually be given dopamine agonists as the initial therapy because motor complications from levodopa are a significant issue for these patients and the dopamine agonists reduce the incidence of motor complications.

- If the patient is above 70 years of age, they will usually be started on levodopa because:

  - older patients are less likely to be affected by motor complications from levodopa
  - levodopa is less likely to cause problems for people with coexisting medical conditions
  - levodopa is better tolerated than most other classes of Parkinson's disease drugs

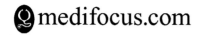

in terms of both cognitive and behavioral side effects
- levodopa is usually used as the initial treatment for any patient who has cognitive impairment

Beyond these general principles, there is a great deal of variation in how patients are medicated. It is crucial for the patient to be under the care of a doctor who has extensive knowledge and experience in the diagnosis and treatment of Parkinson's disease. The decisions to add medications, and to raise or lower doses, are made very carefully and must be monitored by a medical professional who is intimately familiar with the nuances of the progression of Parkinson's disease as well as controlling side effects.

As the disease and level of disability progress, there are several options to manage motor complications that arise. These include:

- Smaller and more frequent doses of levodopa
- Adding or increasing dopamine agonists to levodopa
- Adding MAO-B or COMT inhibitors in order to increase the half-life of levodopa
- Adding amantadine or selegiline to reduce dyskinesia

An article appeared in *Journal of Neurology* in 2008 (vol. 255, supp. 5:pp. 57-59) regarding the initiation of treatment for Parkinson's disease. Some of the observations of the author include:

- Until recently, treatment for PD was initiated at the request of the patient when motor symptoms impaired quality of life. However recent studies have shown that starting medication early yields better long-term results. This author initiates treatment of early PD with an MAOB inhibitor (e.g. rasigiline) and adds a dopamine agonist when motor function begins to decline and bases his approach on three factors:

  - MAOB inhibitors do not cause side effects of dopaminergic drugs such as edema, hypotension and nausea.
  - Recent evidence shows that rasagiline improves bradykinesia, tremor, and rigidity
  - Rasagiline may provide neuroprotection which is important since it is estimated that at the time on onset of PD, up to 40% of dopaminergic neurons are still functioning.

- A study called ELLDOPA (Early vs. Later L-dopa) that was published in 2004 in the *New England Journal of Medicine* (vol. 351:pp. 2498-2508) found that untreated PD patients lost eight points on the PD disability scale during the first ten months after diagnosis, while patients treated with dopaminergic drugs gained six points. This is a significant clinical difference.

- Early treatment with rasagiline or dopamine agonists has been shown to postpone the development of dyskinesia.

- For PD patients that have problems with complex medication schedules, there are three options for once-daily medications including cabergoline (Cabaser), rotigotine patch (Neupro), or slow release formulation of ropinirole (Requip Modutab). (Cabergoline and the rotigotine patch are not available in the U.S.)

To read more about this authors approach to treatment for PD, please click on the following link: http://www.ncbi.nlm.nih.gov/pubmed/18787883

Prognosis for Parkinson's Disease

Parkinson's disease is a chronic, progressive condition that is associated with increasing disability in areas such as motor function, balance, mood, cognition, behavior, activities of daily living, and quality of life. With appropriate treatment, the average life expectancy of the Parkinson's disease patient is considered to be the same as for people who do not suffer from Parkinson's disease; however, complications of advanced Parkinson's disease such as pneumonia, choking, or falling, can lead to earlier mortality. If left untreated, Parkinson's disease progresses to total disability and can be the cause of early death.

The progression of motor symptoms in Parkinson's disease is usually very slow although this can vary widely among patients. Over time, the severity and types of symptoms intensify with some symptoms being related to Parkinson's itself and some related to side effects of medications. With proper treatment, patients can live productive lives for many years.

Studies report that up to 40% of patients with PD develop motor symptoms within four to six years following disease onset. They may appear as abnormal involuntary movements that involve the head, trunk, and limbs, motor fluctuations, and/or an overall decline in motor performance. The development of motor symptoms has been associated with younger age of onset of PD, increased disease severity, and higher doses of levodopa medication. Motor complications generally increase in severity and frequency with increasing duration of PD.

The major challenge for patients with Parkinson's disease is adapting to their progressive disability. With the initial diagnosis of Parkinson's disease, the patient and doctor must determine the level of discomfort or inconvenience of the symptoms in daily life and, based on these findings, establish the initial decisions for therapy. On the average, if initial symptoms are mild, up to three years may pass from the time of diagnosis to the commencement of therapy with levodopa and another three to five years may pass before side effects from the levodopa interfere with daily living. There is no set "timetable" regarding treatment for Parkinson's disease and important issues such as when to start medications, or when to add or change medications, are in part determined by the patient's assessment of the level of interference with daily life that the symptoms present.

Most patients respond to treatment though the extent varies widely among patients. There are several classes of drugs used to treat symptoms and several medications within each class of drugs that can be taken either alone (monotherapy) or as combinations. Successful drug treatment is a delicate balance of correctly dosing medications to achieve relief of symptoms while keeping side-effects at a tolerable level. When medication alone does not provide sufficient relief, there are surgical options available that not only provide relief for eligible patients, but in some cases also lead to lower doses of levodopa.

As symptoms of Parkinson's disease intensify, some patients may require caregiving beyond what family members can provide and may need to investigate the option of professional caregivers or different types of assisted-living arrangements.

The American Academy of Neurology noted in the Practice Guidelines published in 2006 the following points regarding prognosis in PD:

- A rapid rate of decline is associated with:

    - older age at onset (57-78) and rigidity/hypokinesia as an early symptom
    - male gender
    - postural instability
    - gait disorder
    - comorbidities (such as stroke, visual impairment)

- Older age at onset and rigidity at diagnosis "probably" predict earlier cognitive decline and dementia.

- Tremor as an early presenting symptom predicts slow progression of PD, longer response to levodopa, and a relatively good prognosis.
- Dementia, older age at onset, and decreased dopamine responsiveness may predict increased risk of placement in a nursing home as well as shorter survival.

The Role of Alternative Medicine in Parkinson's Disease

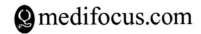

There are increasing numbers of professionals who combine knowledge of conventional treatment of Parkinson's disease with knowledge of complementary medicine. Research in this field is very active. There are limited clinical trials regarding Parkinson's disease and complementary medicine; most information is based on anecdotal evidence. It is important to notify your health care provider if you are using any alternative therapies, no matter how insignificant or benign they may seem.

To see the latest conclusions of the American Academy of Neurology regarding the use of alternative medicine for the treatment of Parkinson's disease, please click on the following link:

http://aan.com/professionals/practice/guidelines/Neuroprotective_PD.pdf

Some forms of complementary medicine related to Parkinson's disease include:

Antioxidants

As noted above, there are ongoing studies regarding *Co-enzyme Q10*, a vitamin-like antioxidant that may have protective benefits for persons with Parkinson's disease. There was also hope that high doses of vitamin E could be protective, however, studies have shown no benefit and some research suggests that some antioxidant vitamins may be harmful in high doses.

Herbal Preparations

- Primrose oil for reducing tremors
- Passionflower for reducing agitation and insomnia
- Ginger for reducing nausea and vomiting from medications
- Milk thistle to enhance liver function by removing toxins from the body

Acupuncture

It has been established that acupuncture causes certain physiological responses in the body that many patients claim brings relief to various Parkinson's disease symptoms. In a pilot study of acupuncture for Parkinson's disease, the only symptom that benefited from acupuncture was reduced sleep disturbance.

Traditional Chinese Medicine

This focuses on establishing balance in the body through treatment of meridians (channels of energy) as well as other modalities.

Massage Therapy

There are several types of massage therapy. Many Parkinson's disease patients report

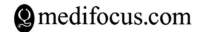

muscle relief as well as other symptomatic relief with this modality of treatment.

Yoga

Yoga promotes relaxation and stretching which some patients with Parkinson's disease find helpful.

Tai Chi

Effective in some Parkinson's disease patients to improve balance by using slow movement to relax and strengthen muscles.

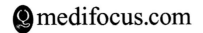

Quality of Life Issues in Parkinson's Disease

The diagnosis and symptoms of Parkinson's disease can be devastating to an individual and family. However, there are several excellent resources available for education and support, and ongoing research has lead to important developments in controlling symptoms and improving quality of life.

Support groups are important because the increasing difficulty of activities of daily life and the progression of symptoms can be demoralizing. Patients and caregivers can benefit from the support of people who understand what they are experiencing and can suggest ways of coping that professionals may not discuss. This also helps reduce the feeling of loneliness that many Parkinson's disease patients and their caregivers may feel.

Dementia is about six times more common in the elderly person with Parkinson's disease than in the average older adult. Support groups can be helpful in coping with dementia. The health care team can provide education and resources for managing difficult or unsafe behaviors that may develop.

Since depression is such a common complication of Parkinson's disease, it is important to seek treatment as soon as possible. In addition to the treatments mentioned above for depression, it is also helpful for the patient to stay socially active and involved with family and friends.

Due to the slow rate of progression on Parkinson's disease, there is ample time for patients and their families or caregivers to focus on future planning for issues such as:

- Contacting an attorney regarding estate planning, will, etc.
- Arranging long-term health/life/disability insurance policies.
- Making adjustments in their professional lives.
- Determining possible modifications to be made in the work environment to facilitate continuing employment.
- Investigating plans for future care, such as professional caregiver, assisted-living facility, or nursing home.

Lifestyle Interventions for Parkinson's Disease and Associated Symptoms

As Parkinson's disease progresses, a multidisciplinary team approach is usually the best approach for maintaining the quality of life of the patient. The team members may include a family doctor, a Parkinson's disease specialist, neurosurgeon, urologist, nurse, social

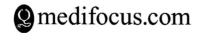

worker, physical therapist, occupational therapist, speech therapist, nutritionist, and, perhaps even complementary medicine professionals, among others.

Lifestyle interventions for Parkinson's disease associated symptoms include:

Problems with Walking

Exercise and physical activity are important in maintaining muscle strength, function and coordination. Physical therapists can teach new methods for standing, turning, and walking that can maximize function and reduce the risk of falling. There are a variety of techniques for managing "freezing" that can significantly improve mobility and safety.

Problems with Drooling

To reduce nighttime drooling, the patient may be helped by sleeping in a more upright position. The patient will also be taught to swallow more frequently than before, especially while eating. In addition, speech therapists can teach the Parkinson's disease patient how to strengthen the muscles used in swallowing.

When the drooling becomes pronounced, some doctors prescribe levodopa or dopamine agonists if not already being used, though their benefit is limited. Anticholinergic drugs may be beneficial but they have several side effects including constipation, urine retention, and cognitive impairments, especially in the older patients.

A drug that is now being evaluated to reduce drooling is botulinum toxin (Botox) which is injected into each parotid gland (the gland that produces saliva in the base of the mouth). Preliminary studies indicate that Botox injections decrease drooling for several weeks.

Speech Problems

A speech therapist is very helpful in evaluating and implementing techniques and suggestions for optimizing voice and speech function. Issues such as hurried speech and soft voice can all be addressed. The therapist can also coach the patient and suggest methods to improve communication.

Some patients undergo an experimental procedure where collagen is injected into the vocal folds of the larynx to enhance vocal quality.

Depression

There are several avenues to helping the Parkinson's disease patient diagnosed with depression. Among these are:

- Counseling in individual or group therapy sessions.
- Consultation with a social worker or psychologist/psychiatrist who may be able to

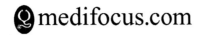

help identify sources of stress and anxiety and help make changes and readjustments in everyday life to reduce them.

- Exercise (e.g., walking) or other physical activity which not only impacts depression but has the added benefit of alleviating motor complications in some patients.
- Medications - The most commonly used antidepressants are selective serotonin reuptake inhibitors (SSRIs) and tricyclic antidepressants (TCAs). Some doctors prefer SSRIs because they are tolerated easily and do not affect mood or memory. TCAs cause orthostatic hypotension (drop in blood pressure when in standing position) in some patients and have more side effects (e.g., dry mouth, blurred vision, and cognitive impairment). They also can be dangerous for patients with certain cardiac conditions.

Some studies suggest that the dopamine agonist *pramipexole* is also effective for treating depression in Parkinson's disease and some doctors prefer to try this drug before suggesting antidepressants.

Pain

Pain in PD is a significant problem and is treated by pinpointing whenever possible the source of the pain. Treatment may include introducing dopamine agonists, modifying the dose of medication that the patient may already be taking, the use of pain killers or antidepressants, or deep brain stimulation.

Sleep Disturbances

Since sleep disturbances may be related to Parkinson's disease medications, the doctor may adjust dosages or even change medications. If the patient has problems with excessive daytime sleepiness, the doctor may prescribe a stimulant.

There are also modifications that can be made in the patient's sleeping environment. These include:

- Use of satin sheets which are smooth and may make it easier for the patient with stiffness to move or get comfortable in bed.
- Using well-placed pillows to help sleepers stay in a comfortable position and prevent them from rolling back into an uncomfortable position.

It is important to discuss any changes in sleep patterns with your doctor since lack of restful sleep can cause significant interference in daytime and nighttime quality of life, not only for the patient with Parkinson's disease but also for the caregiver. The caregiver needs to get an adequate amount of sleep to remain strong and supportive. Rehabilitation professionals should be able to make suggestions to help the caregiver in this area.

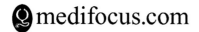

Constipation

This problem may be alleviated by ensuring that the Parkinson's disease patient drinks adequate amounts of fluids and eats a high-fiber diet of fruits and vegetables.

Frequent Urination

A urologist is helpful in evaluating this disorder and suggesting effective treatments. The doctor must determine if the problem is due to medications, infection, comorbid symptoms of aging (e.g., enlarged prostate), or multi-system atrophy (Shy-Drager Syndrome) which shares many similar symptoms with Parkinson's disease such as slow movement, stiff muscles, and mild tremors. There are medications and modifications in daily life that can be suggested for addressing bladder issues as PD progresses.

Weight Loss

Since Parkinson's disease patients are particularly at risk for weight loss, it is important to take steps to manage this issue. Weight loss is partially related to problems that develop with muscles involved in swallowing and makes eating more difficult. Modifications can be made by a speech therapist who may be able to help the patient optimize muscle control or a nutritionist who can teach the patient to modify eating habits so the greatest nutritive benefit is gained.

Helpful suggestions may include:

- Supplementing meals with high calorie drinks
- Frequent small meals
- Modifying the consistency of foods given to the patient to minimize choking or coughing

Since thirst normally diminishes with age and PD medications can cause dehydration, it is critical for patients to focus on drinking adequate amounts of water.

Shortness of Breath

Shortness of breath may be partially controlled by modifying dosage and scheduling of Parkinson's disease medications. Physical therapy is also important in order for the patient to optimize tone and flexibility of the chest muscles.

Visual Disturbances

Modification of the environment may help minimize disturbances of vision. Some suggestions include:

- Brighter lights
- Greater contrast of color between floor and furniture

- Greater contrast where there are changes on the floor (e.g., steps, rugs, etc.)

New Developments

- In August 2009, the U.S. Food and Drug Administration (FDA) notified the public that companies that manufacture pergolide (Permax) agreed to withdraw the drug from the market due to the potential for a serious side effect of heart valve damage.

- Scientists are investigating alternative methods for delivering levodopa, thus avoiding many of the side effects that come with the fluctuation of levels of orally administered levodopa in the blood. Among the techniques being studied are implantable pumps which provide a continuous controlled supply of levodopa. Other models being investigated include medicated skin patches and implanting capsules of dopamine-producing cells into the brain. To read more about drug delivery systems that are used and that are under development, please click on the following link: http://www.ncbi.nlm.nih.gov/pubmed/19651197

- Investigators are studying the feasibility of genetically engineering cells (e.g., skin cells) that can be grown in the laboratory to produce dopamine and then implanting them into the brains of patients with Parkinson's disease. A great advantage would be that cells would be readily available and also that the cells would be obtained from the Parkinson's disease patient, thereby eliminating the problem of immune rejection. To read more about this exciting development, please click on the following link: http://journals.lww.com/neurotodayonline/Fulltext/2009/04160/PD*Patients*_Skin*Cells*Reprogrammed*Into*Stem.1.aspx

- One of the areas of Parkinson's research that receiving considerable attention is that of neuroprotection of brain cells that would slow down the progression of the disease or perhaps even stop its progression. To read more about neuroprotective agents for PD, please click on the following link: http://www.ncbi.nlm.nih.gov/pubmed/19772974

- Researchers are investigating a new technique called *dorsal column stimulation* as an alternative to deep brain stimulation for the treatment of PD symptoms. The research is currently in early stages and is not yet being tested on humans but appears to be promising. The National Institute of Neurological Disorders and Stroke (NINDS) published a description of *dorsal column stimulation* research at the following link: http://www.ninds.nih.gov/newsand*events/news*articles/news*dcsparkinson*rats.htm

- Researchers reported that five late stage Parkinson's disease patients showed significant improvement when the protein *GDNF* was introduced into the *putamen* area of the brain (which regulates movement) by a tube connected to a mini-pump. It reduced "off" time and reduced or eliminated dyskinesia. Some researchers see this exciting development as a potential vehicle to treat the underlying disease in addition to symptoms. This drug is still in very early stages of development and testing.

- There is active investigation of the possible link between *statins* (cholesterol lowering drugs) and neuroprotection in Parkinson's disease. Results from various studies regarding this relationship are not consistent. For more information about statins and PD, you can click on the following link:
  http://www.ncbi.nlm.nih.gov/pubmed/19366342

- Trials of new medications intended to slow the progression of Parkinson's disease are currently underway. Information regarding ongoing clinical studies in your area can be obtained at the Clinical Trials Listing Service at http://www.centerwatch.com or at http://www.clincialtrials.gov

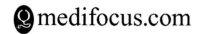medifocus.com

Questions to Ask Your Doctor about Parkinson's Disease

- What is my stage of Parkinson's and what treatments are appropriate at this stage?
- What follow-up is necessary?
- Do I have to restrict or change my daily routine?
- How will Parkinson's disease affect my employment?
- How should I prepare my employer for the changes that will have to be made to accommodate my disability?
- What diet and exercise regime should I follow?
- At what point should I begin taking medication?
- Which medication is most appropriate for my symptoms?
- What side effects should I anticipate from the medication?
- At what point should I consider surgery?
- Will complementary medicine help my symptoms at the present stage?
- Who will assemble the team of allied health professionals that I will need and coordinate my care?
- What is the prognosis (outlook) for short and long-term?
- What resources are available to me and my family for education and support?
- Are there any clinical trials in which it would be appropriate for me to participate?

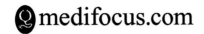

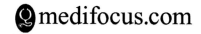 medifocus.com

NOTES

Use this page for taking notes as you review your Guidebook

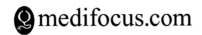

3 - Guide to the Medical Literature

Introduction

This section of your *MediFocus Guidebook* is a comprehensive bibliography of important recent medical literature published about the condition from authoritative, trustworthy medical journals. This is the same information that is used by physicians and researchers to keep up with the latest advances in clinical medicine and biomedical research. A broad spectrum of articles is included in each *MediFocus Guidebook* to provide information about standard treatments, treatment options, new developments, and advances in research.

To facilitate your review and analysis of this information, the articles in this *MediFocus Guidebook* are grouped in the following categories:

- Review Articles - 58 Articles
- General Interest Articles - 58 Articles
- Drug Therapy Articles - 3 Articles
- Clinical Trials Articles - 59 Articles
- Deep Brain Stimulation Articles - 11 Articles

The following information is provided for each of the articles referenced in this section of your *MediFocus Guidebook:*

- Title of the article
- Name of the authors
- Institution where the study was done
- Journal reference (Volume, page numbers, year of publication)
- Link to Abstract (brief summary of the actual article)

Linking to Abstracts: Most of the medical journal articles referenced in this section of your *MediFocus Guidebook* include an abstract (brief summary of the actual article) that can be accessed online via the National Library of Medicine's PubMed® database. You can easily access the individual article abstracts online by entering the individual URL address for a particular article into your web browser, or by going to the following special URL:

http://www.medifocus.com/links/NR013/0112

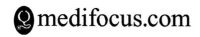

Recent Literature: What Your Doctor Reads

Database: PubMed <June 2009 to January 2012>

Review Articles

1.

Does vigorous exercise have a neuroprotective effect in Parkinson disease?

Author:	Ahlskog JE
Institution:	Department of Neurology, Mayo Clinic, Rochester, MN 55905, USA. eahlskog@mayo.edu
Journal:	Neurology. 2011 Jul 19;77(3):288-94.
Abstract Link:	http://www.medifocus.com/abstracts.php?gid=NR013&ID=21768599

2.

Treatment of depressive symptoms in Parkinson's disease.

Author:	Barone P
Institution:	Department of Neurological Sciences, University of Napoli Federico II-IDC Hermitage Capodimonte, Naples, Italy. barone@unina.it
Journal:	Eur J Neurol. 2011 Mar;18 Suppl 1:11-5. doi: 10.1111/j.1468-1331.2010.03325.x.
Abstract Link:	http://www.medifocus.com/abstracts.php?gid=NR013&ID=21255198

3.

Gene therapy: a viable therapeutic strategy for Parkinson's disease?

Authors:	Berry AL; Foltynie T
Institution:	Department of Molecular Neuroscience, UCL Institute of Neurology, Queen Square, London, WC1N 3BG, UK.
Journal:	J Neurol. 2011 Feb;258(2):179-88. Epub 2010 Oct 21.
Abstract Link:	http://www.medifocus.com/abstracts.php?gid=NR013&ID=20963433

Go to http://www.medifocus.com/links/NR013/0112 for direct online access to the above Abstract Links.

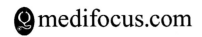

4.

Deep brain stimulation for Parkinson disease: an expert consensus and review of key issues.

Authors:	Bronstein JM; Tagliati M; Alterman RL; Lozano AM; Volkmann J; Stefani A; Horak FB; Okun MS; Foote KD; Krack P; Pahwa R; Henderson JM; Hariz MI; Bakay RA; Rezai A; Marks WJ Jr; Moro E; Vitek JL; Weaver FM; Gross RE; DeLong MR
Institution:	University of California, Los Angeles, School of Medicine, Department of Neurology, 710 Westwood Plaza, Los Angeles, CA 90095, USA. jbronste@ucla.edu
Journal:	Arch Neurol. 2011 Feb;68(2):165. Epub 2010 Oct 11.
Abstract Link:	http://www.medifocus.com/abstracts.php?gid=NR013&ID=20937936

5.

The contributions of antioxidant activity of lipoic acid in reducing neurogenerative progression of Parkinson's disease: a review.

Authors:	De Araujo DP; Lobato Rde F; Cavalcanti JR; Sampaio LR; Araujo PV; Silva MC; Neves KR; Fonteles MM; Sousa FC; Vasconcelos SM
Institution:	Department of Physiology and Pharmacology, Faculty of Medicine, Federal University of Ceara, Brazil.
Journal:	Int J Neurosci. 2011 Feb;121(2):51-7. Epub 2010 Dec 2.
Abstract Link:	http://www.medifocus.com/abstracts.php?gid=NR013&ID=21126109

6.

Statins--increasing or reducing the risk of Parkinson's disease?

Authors:	Dolga AM; Culmsee C; de Lau L; Winter Y; Oertel WH; Luiten PG; Eisel UL
Institution:	Institut fur Pharmakologie und Klinische Pharmazie, Philipps-Universitat Marburg, Germany.
Journal:	Exp Neurol. 2011 Mar;228(1):1-4. Epub 2010 Nov 24.
Abstract Link:	**ABSTRACT NOT AVAILABLE**

Go to http://www.medifocus.com/links/NR013/0112 for direct online access to the above Abstract Links.

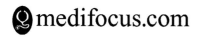

7.

Deep brain stimulation for Parkinson's disease, essential tremor, and dystonia.

Author:	Eller T
Institution:	NorthShore University HealthSystem, Evanston Hospital, Evanston, Illinois, USA.
Journal:	Dis Mon. 2011 Oct;57(10):638-46.
Abstract Link:	**ABSTRACT NOT AVAILABLE**

8.

Gender distribution of patients with Parkinson's disease treated with subthalamic deep brain stimulation; a review of the 2000-2009 literature.

Authors:	Hariz GM; Nakajima T; Limousin P; Foltynie T; Zrinzo L; Jahanshahi M; Hamberg K
Institution:	Department of Community Medicine and Rehabilitation, Occupational Therapy, University of Umea, Sweden. gun-marie.hariz@neuro.umu.se
Journal:	Parkinsonism Relat Disord. 2011 Mar;17(3):146-9. Epub 2010 Dec 30.
Abstract Link:	http://www.medifocus.com/abstracts.php?gid=NR013&ID=21195012

9.

Excessive daytime sleepiness in patients with Parkinson's disease.

Authors:	Knie B; Mitra MT; Logishetty K; Chaudhuri KR
Institution:	Charit Universitatsmedizin Berlin, Berlin, Germany.
Journal:	CNS Drugs. 2011 Mar 1;25(3):203-12. doi: 10.2165/11539720-000000000-00000.
Abstract Link:	http://www.medifocus.com/abstracts.php?gid=NR013&ID=21323392

Go to http://www.medifocus.com/links/NR013/0112 for direct online access to the above Abstract Links.

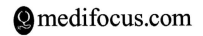

10.

The role of dopamine agonists in the treatment of depression in patients with Parkinson's disease: a systematic review.

Author:	Leentjens AF
Institution:	Department of Psychiatry, Maastricht University Medical Centre, Maastricht, the Netherlands. a.leentjens@maastrichtuniversity.nl
Journal:	Drugs. 2011 Feb 12;71(3):273-86. doi: 10.2165/11585380-000000000-00000.
Abstract Link:	http://www.medifocus.com/abstracts.php?gid=NR013&ID=21319866

11.

Meta-analysis of the relationship between Parkinson disease and melanoma.

Authors:	Liu R; Gao X; Lu Y; Chen H
Institution:	Epidemiology Branch, National Institute of Environmental Health Sciences, Research Triangle Park, NC 27709, USA.
Journal:	Neurology. 2011 Jun 7;76(23):2002-9.
Abstract Link:	http://www.medifocus.com/abstracts.php?gid=NR013&ID=21646627

12.

New non-oral drug delivery systems for Parkinson's disease treatment.

Authors:	Md S; Haque S; Sahni JK; Baboota S; Ali J
Institution:	Department of Pharmaceutics, Faculty of Pharmacy, Jamia Hamdard, Hamdard Nagar, New Delhi 110062, India.
Journal:	Expert Opin Drug Deliv. 2011 Mar;8(3):359-74. Epub 2011 Feb 12.
Abstract Link:	http://www.medifocus.com/abstracts.php?gid=NR013&ID=21314492

Go to http://www.medifocus.com/links/NR013/0112 for direct online access to the above Abstract Links.

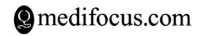

13.

Therapeutic role of 5-HT1A receptors in the treatment of schizophrenia and Parkinson's disease.

Author:	Ohno Y
Institution:	Laboratory of Pharmacology, Osaka University of Pharmaceutical Sciences, Nasahara, Takatsuki, Osaka, Japan. yohno@gly.oups.ac.jp
Journal:	CNS Neurosci Ther. 2011 Feb;17(1):58-65. doi: 10.1111/j.1755-5949.2010.00211.x. Epub 2010 Nov 21.
Abstract Link:	http://www.medifocus.com/abstracts.php?gid=NR013&ID=21091640

14.

The association between Parkinson's disease and melanoma.

Authors:	Pan T; Li X; Jankovic J
Institution:	Diana Helis Henry Medical Research Foundation, New Orleans, LA, USA.
Journal:	Int J Cancer. 2011 May 15;128(10):2251-60. doi: 10.1002/ijc.25912. Epub 2011 Mar 14.
Abstract Link:	http://www.medifocus.com/abstracts.php?gid=NR013&ID=21207412

15.

Gastrointestinal dysfunction in Parkinson's disease.

Author:	Pfeiffer RF
Institution:	Department of Neurology, University of Tennessee Health Science Center, 855 Monroe Avenue, Memphis, TN 38163, USA. rpfeiffer@uthsc.edu
Journal:	Parkinsonism Relat Disord. 2011 Jan;17(1):10-5. Epub 2010 Sep 15.
Abstract Link:	http://www.medifocus.com/abstracts.php?gid=NR013&ID=20829091

Go to http://www.medifocus.com/links/NR013/0112 for direct online access to the above Abstract Links.

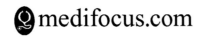

16.

Drugs and drug delivery in PD: optimizing control of symptoms with pramipexole prolonged-release.

Author: Rascol O

Institution: Department of Clinical Pharmacology and Neurosciences, INSERM U825 and Clinical Investigation Center, University Hospital, Toulouse, France. rascol@cict.fr

Journal: Eur J Neurol. 2011 Mar;18 Suppl 1:3-10. doi: 10.1111/j.1468-1331.2010.03326.x.

Abstract Link: http://www.medifocus.com/abstracts.php?gid=NR013&ID=21255197

17.

Determinants of health-related quality of life in Parkinson's disease: a systematic review.

Authors: Soh SE; Morris ME; McGinley JL

Institution: Melbourne School of Health Sciences, The University of Melbourne, 200 Berkeley Street, Victoria 3010, Australia. ssoh@unimelb.edu.au

Journal: Parkinsonism Relat Disord. 2011 Jan;17(1):1-9. Epub 2010 Sep 15.

Abstract Link: http://www.medifocus.com/abstracts.php?gid=NR013&ID=20833572

18.

Cell transplantation and gene therapy in Parkinson's disease.

Authors: Wakeman DR; Dodiya HB; Kordower JH

Journal: Mt Sinai J Med. 2011 Jan-Feb;78(1):126-58. doi: 10.1002/msj.20233.

Abstract Link: http://www.medifocus.com/abstracts.php?gid=NR013&ID=21259269

Go to http://www.medifocus.com/links/NR013/0112 for direct online access to the above Abstract Links.

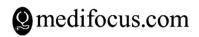

19.

Preclinical biomarkers of Parkinson disease.

Authors: Wu Y; Le W; Jankovic J
Institution: Department of Neurology, Shanghai First People's Hospital, Shanghai
                 Jiao Tong University School of Medicine, Shanghai, China.
Journal: Arch Neurol. 2011 Jan;68(1):22-30.
Abstract Link: http://www.medifocus.com/abstracts.php?gid=NR013&ID=21220674

20.

Oral and infusion levodopa-based strategies for managing motor complications in patients with Parkinson's disease.

Authors: Antonini A; Chaudhuri KR; Martinez-Martin P; Odin P
Institution: IRRCS, San Camillo, Viale Alberoni 70, Venice, Italy.
                 angelo3000@yahoo.com
Journal: CNS Drugs. 2010 Feb 1;24(2):119-29. doi:
                 10.2165/11310940-000000000-00000.
Abstract Link: http://www.medifocus.com/abstracts.php?gid=NR013&ID=20088619

21.

Role of pramipexole in the management of Parkinson's disease.

Authors: Antonini A; Barone P; Ceravolo R; Fabbrini G; Tinazzi M;
                 Abbruzzese G
Institution: Department for Parkinson Disease, IRCCS San Camillo, Venice, Italy.
                 angelo3000@yahoo.com
Journal: CNS Drugs. 2010 Oct 1;24(10):829-41. doi:
                 10.2165/11585090-000000000-00000.
Abstract Link: http://www.medifocus.com/abstracts.php?gid=NR013&ID=20839895

Go to http://www.medifocus.com/links/NR013/0112 for direct online access to the above Abstract Links.

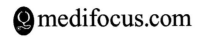

22.

Parkinson's disease and cancer risk: a systematic review and meta-analysis.

Authors: Bajaj A; Driver JA; Schernhammer ES

Institution: Channing Laboratory, Department of Medicine, Brigham and Women's Hospital and Harvard Medical School, 181 Longwood Avenue, Boston, MA 02115, USA. n2baj@channing.harvard.edu

Journal: Cancer Causes Control. 2010 May;21(5):697-707. Epub 2010 Jan 7.

Abstract Link: http://www.medifocus.com/abstracts.php?gid=NR013&ID=20054708

23.

Strategies for treatment of gait and posture associated deficits in movement disorders: the impact of deep brain stimulation.

Authors: Botzel K; Kraft E

Institution: Department of Neurology, University Hospital, Ludwig-Maximilian-University, 81366 Munich, Germany. kBotzel@med.uni-muenchen.de

Journal: Restor Neurol Neurosci. 2010;28(1):115-22.

Abstract Link: http://www.medifocus.com/abstracts.php?gid=NR013&ID=20086288

24.

Is there muscular weakness in Parkinson's disease?

Authors: Cano-de-la-Cuerda R; Perez-de-Heredia M; Miangolarra-Page JC; Munoz-Hellin E; Fernandez-de-Las-Penas C

Institution: Department of Physical Therapy, Occupational Therapy, Physical Medicine and Rehabilitation, Universidad Rey Juan Carlos, Alcorcon, Madrid, Spain.

Journal: Am J Phys Med Rehabil. 2010 Jan;89(1):70-6.

Abstract Link: http://www.medifocus.com/abstracts.php?gid=NR013&ID=19487924

Go to http://www.medifocus.com/links/NR013/0112 for direct online access to the above Abstract Links.

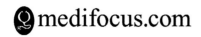

25.

Pramipexole extended release: in Parkinson's disease.

Authors:	Chwieduk CM; Curran MP
Institution:	Adis, a Wolters Kluwer Business, North Shore, Auckland, New Zealand. demail@adis.co.nz
Journal:	CNS Drugs. 2010 Apr;24(4):327-36. doi: 10.2165/11204570-000000000-00000.
Abstract Link:	http://www.medifocus.com/abstracts.php?gid=NR013&ID=20297857

26.

Parkinson's disease dementia.

Authors:	Docherty MJ; Burn DJ
Institution:	Institute for Ageing and Health, Newcastle University, Newcastle upon Tyne, UK.
Journal:	Curr Neurol Neurosci Rep. 2010 Jul;10(4):292-8.
Abstract Link:	http://www.medifocus.com/abstracts.php?gid=NR013&ID=20428976

27.

Emerging parkinsonian phenotypes.

Authors:	Elia AE; Albanese A
Institution:	Fondazione, IRCCS Istituto Neurologico Carlo Besta, Universita Cattolica del Sacro Cuore, Via G. Celoria 11, 20133 Milano, Italy.
Journal:	Rev Neurol (Paris). 2010 Oct;166(10):834-40.
Abstract Link:	http://www.medifocus.com/abstracts.php?gid=NR013&ID=20817231

Go to http://www.medifocus.com/links/NR013/0112 for direct online access to the above Abstract Links.

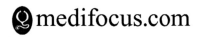

28.

Management of hallucinations and psychosis in Parkinson's disease.

Authors:	Eng ML; Welty TE
Institution:	Department of Pharmacy Practice, University of Kansas School of Pharmacy, Kansas City, Kansas 66160, USA. meng@kumc.edu
Journal:	Am J Geriatr Pharmacother. 2010 Aug;8(4):316-30.
Abstract Link:	http://www.medifocus.com/abstracts.php?gid=NR013&ID=20869621

29.

Management of motor complications in Parkinson disease: current and emerging therapies.

Author:	Espay AJ
Institution:	Department of Neurology, James J. and Joan A. Gardner Center for Parkinson's disease and Movement Disorders, University of Cincinnati Neuroscience Institute, 260 Stetson Street, Suite 2300, PO Box 670525, Cincinnati, OH 45267-0525, USA. alberto.espay@uc.edu
Journal:	Neurol Clin. 2010 Nov;28(4):913-25.
Abstract Link:	http://www.medifocus.com/abstracts.php?gid=NR013&ID=20816270

30.

Surgical management of Parkinson's disease.

Authors:	Foltynie T; Hariz MI
Institution:	UCL Institute of Neurology, Queen Square, London, UK. t.foltynie@ion.ucl.ac.uk
Journal:	Expert Rev Neurother. 2010 Jun;10(6):903-14.
Abstract Link:	http://www.medifocus.com/abstracts.php?gid=NR013&ID=20518607

Go to http://www.medifocus.com/links/NR013/0112 for direct online access to the above Abstract Links.

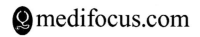
31.

Anti-inflammatory drugs and risk of Parkinson disease: a meta-analysis.

Authors:	Gagne JJ; Power MC
Institution:	Department of Epidemiology, Harvard School of Public Health, Boston, MA, USA. jgagne1@partners.org
Journal:	Neurology. 2010 Mar 23;74(12):995-1002.
Abstract Link:	http://www.medifocus.com/abstracts.php?gid=NR013&ID=20308684

32.

Manganese and Parkinson's disease: a critical review and new findings.

Author:	Guilarte TR
Institution:	Neurotoxicology and Molecular Imaging Laboratory, Department of Environmental Health Sciences, Johns Hopkins Bloomberg School of Public Health, Baltimore, Maryland, USA. trguilarte@columbia.edu
Journal:	Environ Health Perspect. 2010 Aug;118(8):1071-80. Epub 2010 Apr 19.
Abstract Link:	http://www.medifocus.com/abstracts.php?gid=NR013&ID=20403794

33.

The progression of pathology in Parkinson's disease.

Authors:	Halliday GM; McCann H
Institution:	Prince of Wales Medical Research Institute and University of New South Wales, Sydney, Australia. g.halliday@powmri.edu.au
Journal:	Ann N Y Acad Sci. 2010 Jan;1184:188-95.
Abstract Link:	http://www.medifocus.com/abstracts.php?gid=NR013&ID=20146698

Go to http://www.medifocus.com/links/NR013/0112 for direct online access to the above Abstract Links.

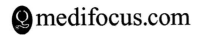

34.

Narcolepsy in Parkinson's disease.

Authors: Haq IZ; Naidu Y; Reddy P; Chaudhuri KR
Institution: Guy's, King's & St Thomas' School of Medicine, King's College, London, UK.
Journal: Expert Rev Neurother. 2010 Jun;10(6):879-84.
Abstract Link: http://www.medifocus.com/abstracts.php?gid=NR013&ID=20518604

35.

Nonmotor symptoms in genetic Parkinson disease.

Authors: Kasten M; Kertelge L; Bruggemann N; van der Vegt J; Schmidt A; Tadic V; Buhmann C; Steinlechner S; Behrens MI; Ramirez A; Binkofski F; Siebner H; Raspe H; Hagenah J; Lencer R; Klein C
Institution: Department of Neurology, University of Lubeck, Lubeck, Germany.
Journal: Arch Neurol. 2010 Jun;67(6):670-6.
Abstract Link: http://www.medifocus.com/abstracts.php?gid=NR013&ID=20558386

36.

Tolerability and safety of ropinirole versus other dopamine agonists and levodopa in the treatment of Parkinson's disease: meta-analysis of randomized controlled trials.

Authors: Kulisevsky J; Pagonabarraga J
Institution: Unit of Movement Disorders, Neurology Department, Hospital de la Santa Creu i Sant Pau, Barcelona, Spain.
Journal: Drug Saf. 2010;33(2):147-61. doi: 10.2165/11319860-000000000-00000.
Abstract Link: http://www.medifocus.com/abstracts.php?gid=NR013&ID=20082541

Go to http://www.medifocus.com/links/NR013/0112 for direct online access to the above Abstract Links.

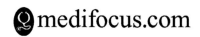

37.

The physical, social and emotional effects of bowel dysfunction in Parkinson's disease.

Author: Kyle G

Institution: Thames Valley University.

Journal: Nurs Times. 2010 Aug 24-30;106(33):20-2.

Abstract Link: http://www.medifocus.com/abstracts.php?gid=NR013&ID=20863022

38.

The role of rasagiline in the treatment of Parkinson's disease.

Authors: Leegwater-Kim J; Bortan E

Institution: Department of Neurology, Tufts University School of Medicine, Lahey
                   Clinic, Burlington, MA 01805, USA. leegwa00@lahey.org

Journal: Clin Interv Aging. 2010 May 25;5:149-56.

Abstract Link: http://www.medifocus.com/abstracts.php?gid=NR013&ID=20517484

39.

Novel anti-inflammatory and neuroprotective agents for Parkinson's disease.

Authors: Lu L; Li F; Wang X

Institution: Department of Physiology, Capital Medical University, Youanmen,
                   Beijing, PR China.

Journal: CNS Neurol Disord Drug Targets. 2010 Apr;9(2):232-40.

Abstract Link: http://www.medifocus.com/abstracts.php?gid=NR013&ID=20015029

Go to http://www.medifocus.com/links/NR013/0112 for direct online access to the above Abstract Links.

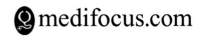

40.

Total knee arthroplasty and Parkinson disease: enhancing outcomes and avoiding complications.

Authors: Macaulay W; Geller JA; Brown AR; Cote LJ; Kiernan HA
Institution: Department of Orthopaedic Surgery, Center for Hip and Knee Replacement, New York-Presbyterian Hospital at Columbia University Medical Center, New York, NY, USA.
Journal: J Am Acad Orthop Surg. 2010 Nov;18(11):687-94.
Abstract Link: http://www.medifocus.com/abstracts.php?gid=NR013&ID=21041803

41.

Dysphagia in Parkinson's disease: a therapeutic challenge?

Authors: Michou E; Hamdy S
Institution: University of Manchester, Salford, UK.
Journal: Expert Rev Neurother. 2010 Jun;10(6):875-8.
Abstract Link: http://www.medifocus.com/abstracts.php?gid=NR013&ID=20518603

42.

Restless Legs Syndrome (RLS) and Parkinson's disease (PD)-related disorders or different entities?

Authors: Moller JC; Unger M; Stiasny-Kolster K; Oertel WH
Institution: Department of Neurology, Philipps-University, Marburg, Germany. carsten.moeller@med.uni-marburg.de
Journal: J Neurol Sci. 2010 Feb 15;289(1-2):135-7. Epub 2009 Sep 15.
Abstract Link: http://www.medifocus.com/abstracts.php?gid=NR013&ID=19755200

Go to http://www.medifocus.com/links/NR013/0112 for direct online access to the above Abstract Links.

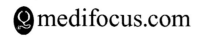

43.

Current understanding and management of Parkinson disease: five new things.

Authors: Morley JF; Hurtig HI

Institution: Parkinson's Disease and Movement Disorders Center, Department of Neurology, University of Pennsylvania, Philadelphia, PA 19107, USA.

Journal: Neurology. 2010 Nov 2;75(18 Suppl 1):S9-15.

Abstract Link: **ABSTRACT NOT AVAILABLE**

44.

Surgical approaches to treatment of Parkinson's disease: Implications for speech function.

Author: Murdoch BE

Institution: The University of Queensland, Brisbane, Australia.
b.murdoch@uq.edu.au

Journal: Int J Speech Lang Pathol. 2010 Oct;12(5):375-84.

Abstract Link: http://www.medifocus.com/abstracts.php?gid=NR013&ID=20602579

45.

Defining disease-modifying therapies for PD--a road map for moving forward.

Authors: Olanow CW; Kieburtz K

Institution: Department of Neurology and Neuroscience, Mount Sinai School of Medicine, New York, New York 10029, USA.
warren.olanow@mssm.edu

Journal: Mov Disord. 2010 Sep 15;25(12):1774-9.

Abstract Link: http://www.medifocus.com/abstracts.php?gid=NR013&ID=20839307

Go to http://www.medifocus.com/links/NR013/0112 for direct online access to the above Abstract Links.

46.

Genitourinary dysfunction in Parkinson's disease.

Authors: Sakakibara R; Uchiyama T; Yamanishi T; Kishi M
Institution: Neurology Division, Department of Internal Medicine, Sakura Medical
                     Center, Toho University, Shimoshizu, Sakura 285-8741, Japan.
                     sakakibara@sakura.med.toho-u.ac.jp
Journal: Mov Disord. 2010 Jan 15;25(1):2-12.
Abstract Link: http://www.medifocus.com/abstracts.php?gid=NR013&ID=20077468

47.

When does Parkinson disease start?

Authors: Savica R; Rocca WA; Ahlskog JE
Institution: Department of Health Sciences Research, Mayo Clinic, Rochester, MN
                     55905, USA.
Journal: Arch Neurol. 2010 Jul;67(7):798-801.
Abstract Link: http://www.medifocus.com/abstracts.php?gid=NR013&ID=20625084

48.

Classifying risk factors for dyskinesia in Parkinson's disease.

Authors: Sharma JC; Bachmann CG; Linazasoro G
Institution: Consultant Physician and Honorary Professor, Sherwood Forest
                     hospitals NHS Trust, University of Nottingham, UK.
                     jagsharma@tiscali.co.uk
Journal: Parkinsonism Relat Disord. 2010 Sep;16(8):490-7. Epub 2010 Jul 3.
Abstract Link: http://www.medifocus.com/abstracts.php?gid=NR013&ID=20598622

Go to http://www.medifocus.com/links/NR013/0112 for direct online access to the above Abstract Links.

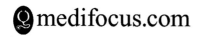
49.

Evaluation of the efficacy and safety of adjuvant treatment to levodopa therapy in Parkinson s disease patients with motor complications.

Authors:	Stowe R; Ives N; Clarke CE; Deane K; Wheatley K; Gray R; Handley K; Furmston A
Institution:	Birmingham Clinical Trials Unit, University of Birmingham, Edgbaston, Birmingham, UK, B15 2TT.
Journal:	Cochrane Database Syst Rev. 2010 Jul 7;7:CD007166.
Abstract Link:	http://www.medifocus.com/abstracts.php?gid=NR013&ID=20614454

50.

Parkinson's disease: oxidative stress and therapeutic approaches.

Authors:	Surendran S; Rajasankar S
Institution:	School of Medicine, LSUHSC, New Orleans, LA 70112, USA. sankar_surendran@yahoo.com
Journal:	Neurol Sci. 2010 Oct;31(5):531-40. Epub 2010 Mar 10.
Abstract Link:	http://www.medifocus.com/abstracts.php?gid=NR013&ID=20221655

51.

Clinical review and treatment of select adverse effects of dopamine receptor agonists in Parkinson's disease.

Author:	Wood LD
Institution:	Department of Pharmacotherapy, College of Pharmacy, Washington State University, Spokane, Washington 99217-6131, USA. lindy_wood@wsu.edu
Journal:	Drugs Aging. 2010 Apr 1;27(4):295-310. doi: 10.2165/11318330-000000000-00000.
Abstract Link:	http://www.medifocus.com/abstracts.php?gid=NR013&ID=20359261

Go to http://www.medifocus.com/links/NR013/0112 for direct online access to the above Abstract Links.

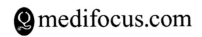

52.

Clinical review of treatment options for select nonmotor symptoms of Parkinson's disease.

Authors:	Wood LD; Neumiller JJ; Setter SM; Dobbins EK
Institution:	Elder Services, Spokane, Washington, USA. lindy_wood@wsu.edu
Journal:	Am J Geriatr Pharmacother. 2010 Aug;8(4):294-315.
Abstract Link:	http://www.medifocus.com/abstracts.php?gid=NR013&ID=20869620

53.

Challenges of treatment adherence in older patients with Parkinson's disease.

Authors:	Bainbridge JL; Ruscin JM
Institution:	Department of Clinical Pharmacy, University of Colorado Denver, Aurora, Colorado 80045, USA. jacci.bainbridge@uchsc.edu
Journal:	Drugs Aging. 2009;26(2):145-55. doi: 10.2165/0002512-200926020-00006.
Abstract Link:	http://www.medifocus.com/abstracts.php?gid=NR013&ID=19220071

54.

Dopamine agonists for early Parkinson disease.

Authors:	Hitzeman N; Rafii F
Institution:	Sutter Health Family Medicine Residency Program, Sacramento, CA, USA. hitzemn@sutterhealth.org
Journal:	Am Fam Physician. 2009 Jul 1;80(1):28-30.
Abstract Link:	http://www.medifocus.com/abstracts.php?gid=NR013&ID=19621842

Go to http://www.medifocus.com/links/NR013/0112 for direct online access to the above Abstract Links.

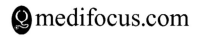

55.

Parkinson's disease.

Authors: Lees AJ; Hardy J; Revesz T

Institution: Department of Molecular Neuroscience and Reta Lila Weston Institute of Neurological Studies, Institute of Neurology, University College London and the National Hospital for Neurology and Neurosurgery, London, UK. alees@ion.ucl.ac.uk

Journal: Lancet. 2009 Jun 13;373(9680):2055-66.

Abstract Link: http://www.medifocus.com/abstracts.php?gid=NR013&ID=19524782

56.

Physical and mental fatigue in Parkinson's disease: epidemiology, pathophysiology and treatment.

Author: Lou JS

Institution: Oregon Health & Science University, Portland, Oregon, USA. Louja@ohsu.edu

Journal: Drugs Aging. 2009;26(3):195-208. doi: 10.2165/00002512-200926030-00002.

Abstract Link: http://www.medifocus.com/abstracts.php?gid=NR013&ID=19358616

57.

Treatment of early Parkinson's disease. Part 1.

Authors: Simuni T; Lyons KE; Pahwa R; Hauser RA; Comella C; Elmer L; Weintraub D

Institution: Department of Neurology, Northwestern University, Parkinson's Disease and Movement Disorders Center, Chicago, Ill 60611, USA. tsimuni@nmff.org

Journal: Eur Neurol. 2009;61(4):193-205. Epub 2009 Jan 29.

Abstract Link: http://www.medifocus.com/abstracts.php?gid=NR013&ID=19176960

Go to http://www.medifocus.com/links/NR013/0112 for direct online access to the above Abstract Links.

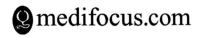
58.

Treatment of early Parkinson's disease. Part 2.

Authors: Simuni T; Lyons KE; Pahwa R; Hauser RA; Comella C; Elmer L;
            Weintraub D

Institution: Department of Neurology, Northwestern University, Parkinson's
            Disease and Movement Disorders Center, Chicago, Ill, USA.
            tsimuni@nmff.org

Journal: Eur Neurol. 2009;61(4):206-15. Epub 2009 Jan 29.
Abstract Link: http://www.medifocus.com/abstracts.php?gid=NR013&ID=19176961

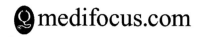

General Interest Articles

59.

Boxing training for patients with Parkinson disease: a case series.

Authors:	Combs SA; Diehl MD; Staples WH; Conn L; Davis K; Lewis N; Schaneman K
Institution:	Krannert School of Physical Therapy, University of Indianapolis, 1400 E Hanna Ave, Indianapolis, IN 46227, USA. scombs@uindy.edu
Journal:	Phys Ther. 2011 Jan;91(1):132-42. Epub 2010 Nov 18.
Abstract Link:	http://www.medifocus.com/abstracts.php?gid=NR013&ID=21088118

60.

Use of ibuprofen and risk of Parkinson disease.

Authors:	Gao X; Chen H; Schwarzschild MA; Ascherio A
Institution:	Channing Laboratory, Department of Medicine, Brigham and Women's Hospital, and Harvard Medical School, 181 Longwood Ave., Boston, MA 02115, USA. xiang.gao@channing.harvard.edu
Journal:	Neurology. 2011 Mar 8;76(10):863-9. Epub 2011 Mar 2.
Abstract Link:	http://www.medifocus.com/abstracts.php?gid=NR013&ID=21368281

61.

Botulinum toxin type A in patients with Parkinson's disease and refractory overactive bladder.

Authors:	Giannantoni A; Conte A; Proietti S; Giovannozzi S; Rossi A; Fabbrini G; Porena M; Berardelli A
Institution:	Department of Urology and Andrology, Ospedale S. Maria della Misericordia, and Department of Neurology, University of Perugia, Perugia, Italy. agianton@libero.it
Journal:	J Urol. 2011 Sep;186(3):960-4. Epub 2011 Jul 24.
Abstract Link:	http://www.medifocus.com/abstracts.php?gid=NR013&ID=21791351

Go to http://www.medifocus.com/links/NR013/0112 for direct online access to the above Abstract Links.

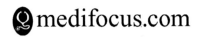

62.

Resting tremor in Parkinson disease: a negative predictor of levodopa-induced dyskinesia.

Authors: Kipfer S; Stephan MA; Schupbach WM; Ballinari P; Kaelin-Lang A

Institution: Movement Disorders Center, Department of Neurology, "Inselspital" Berne University Hospital, University of Berne, Switzerland.

Journal: Arch Neurol. 2011 Aug;68(8):1037-9.

Abstract Link: http://www.medifocus.com/abstracts.php?gid=NR013&ID=21825240

63.

Effect of low-frequency repetitive transcranial magnetic stimulation combined with physical therapy on L-dopa-induced painful off-period dystonia in Parkinson's disease.

Authors: Kodama M; Kasahara T; Hyodo M; Aono K; Sugaya M; Koyama Y; Hanayama K; Masakado Y

Institution: Department of Rehabilitation Medicine, Tokai University School of Medicine, Isehara, Kanagawa, Japan.

Journal: Am J Phys Med Rehabil. 2011 Feb;90(2):150-5.

Abstract Link: http://www.medifocus.com/abstracts.php?gid=NR013&ID=20975525

64.

Limb collapse, rather than instability, causes failure in sit-to-stand performance among patients with parkinson disease.

Authors: Mak MK; Yang F; Pai YC

Institution: Department of Rehabilitation Sciences, The Hong Kong Polytechnic University, Hung Hom, Hong Kong. rsmmak@inet.polyu.edu.hk

Journal: Phys Ther. 2011 Mar;91(3):381-91. Epub 2011 Jan 27.

Abstract Link: http://www.medifocus.com/abstracts.php?gid=NR013&ID=21273628

Go to http://www.medifocus.com/links/NR013/0112 for direct online access to the above Abstract Links.

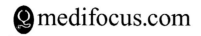

65.

Do co-morbidities and cognition impact functional change and discharge needs in Parkinson disease?

Authors: Marciniak CM; Choo CM; Toledo SD; Semik PE; Aegesen AL

Institution: Northwestern University, Rehabilitation Institute of Chicago, Illinois, USA.

Journal: Am J Phys Med Rehabil. 2011 Apr;90(4):272-80.

Abstract Link: http://www.medifocus.com/abstracts.php?gid=NR013&ID=21765244

66.

Does levodopa accelerate the pathologic process in Parkinson disease brain?

Authors: Parkkinen L; O'Sullivan SS; Kuoppamaki M; Collins C; Kallis C; Holton JL; Williams DR; Revesz T; Lees AJ

Institution: Queen Square Brain Bank for Neurological Disorders, UCL Institute of Neurology, UK.

Journal: Neurology. 2011 Oct 11;77(15):1420-6. Epub 2011 Sep 14.

Abstract Link: http://www.medifocus.com/abstracts.php?gid=NR013&ID=21917769

67.

Vitamin d deficiency-induced vertebral fractures may cause stooped posture in Parkinson disease.

Authors: Sato Y; Iwamoto J; Honda Y

Institution: Department of Neurology, Mitate Hospital, Tagawa, Japan.

Journal: Am J Phys Med Rehabil. 2011 Apr;90(4):281-6.

Abstract Link: http://www.medifocus.com/abstracts.php?gid=NR013&ID=21273899

Go to http://www.medifocus.com/links/NR013/0112 for direct online access to the above Abstract Links.

68.

Profile of functional limitations and task performance among people with early- and middle-stage Parkinson disease.

Authors: Schenkman M; Ellis T; Christiansen C; Baron AE; Tickle-Degnen L; Hall DA; Wagenaar R

Institution: Department of Physical Medicine and Rehabilitation, School of Medicine, University of Colorado, Aurora, CO 80045, USA. margaret.schenkman@ucdenver.edu

Journal: Phys Ther. 2011 Sep;91(9):1339-54. Epub 2011 Jul 21.

Abstract Link: http://www.medifocus.com/abstracts.php?gid=NR013&ID=21778290

69.

Associated factors for REM sleep behavior disorder in Parkinson disease.

Authors: Sixel-Doring F; Trautmann E; Mollenhauer B; Trenkwalder C

Institution: Paracelsus-Elena-Klinik, Center of Parkinsonism and Movement Disorders, Klinikstr. 16, 34128 Kassel, Germany. friederike.sixel@pk-mx.de

Journal: Neurology. 2011 Sep 13;77(11):1048-54. Epub 2011 Aug 10.

Abstract Link: http://www.medifocus.com/abstracts.php?gid=NR013&ID=21832215

70.

Freezing of gait and activity limitations in people with Parkinson's disease.

Authors: Tan DM; McGinley JL; Danoudis ME; Iansek R; Morris ME

Institution: School of Health Sciences, University of Melbourne, Melbourne, Australia. dawn.tan.m.l@sgh.com.sg

Journal: Arch Phys Med Rehabil. 2011 Jul;92(7):1159-65.

Abstract Link: http://www.medifocus.com/abstracts.php?gid=NR013&ID=21704798

Go to http://www.medifocus.com/links/NR013/0112 for direct online access to the above Abstract Links.

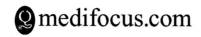

71.

Real-life driving outcomes in Parkinson disease.

Authors:	Uc EY; Rizzo M; Johnson AM; Emerson JL; Liu D; Mills ED; Anderson SW; Dawson JD
Institution:	Department of Neurology, University of Iowa, Carver College of Medicine, Iowa City, IA 52242, USA. ergun-uc@uiowa.edu
Journal:	Neurology. 2011 May 31;76(22):1894-902.
Abstract Link:	http://www.medifocus.com/abstracts.php?gid=NR013&ID=21624988

72.

Olfactory dysfunction, central cholinergic integrity and cognitive impairment in Parkinson's disease.

Authors:	Bohnen NI; Muller ML; Kotagal V; Koeppe RA; Kilbourn MA; Albin RL; Frey KA
Institution:	Department of Radiology, Division of Nuclear Medicine, University of Michigan, Ann Arbor, MI 48109, USA. nbohnen@umich.edu
Journal:	Brain. 2010 Jun;133(Pt 6):1747-54. Epub 2010 Apr 22.
Abstract Link:	http://www.medifocus.com/abstracts.php?gid=NR013&ID=20413575

73.

Smoking duration, intensity, and risk of Parkinson disease.

Authors:	Chen H; Huang X; Guo X; Mailman RB; Park Y; Kamel F; Umbach DM; Xu Q; Hollenbeck A; Schatzkin A; Blair A
Institution:	Epidemiology Branch, National Institute of Environmental Health Sciences, 111 T.W. Alexander Dr., PO Box 12233, Mail drop A3-05, Research Triangle Park, NC 27709, USA. chenh2@niehs.nih.gov
Journal:	Neurology. 2010 Mar 16;74(11):878-84. Epub 2010 Mar 10.
Abstract Link:	http://www.medifocus.com/abstracts.php?gid=NR013&ID=20220126

Go to http://www.medifocus.com/links/NR013/0112 for direct online access to the above Abstract Links.

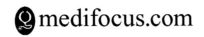

74.

Anxiety disorders in Parkinson's disease: prevalence and risk factors.

Authors: Dissanayaka NN; Sellbach A; Matheson S; O'Sullivan JD; Silburn PA; Byrne GJ; Marsh R; Mellick GD

Institution: Neurology Research Centre, Royal Brisbane and Women's Hospital, Brisbane, Australia. n.dissanayaka@griffith.edu.au

Journal: Mov Disord. 2010 May 15;25(7):838-45.

Abstract Link: http://www.medifocus.com/abstracts.php?gid=NR013&ID=20461800

75.

Gait training with progressive external auditory cueing in persons with Parkinson's disease.

Authors: Ford MP; Malone LA; Nyikos I; Yelisetty R; Bickel CS

Institution: Department of Physical Therapy, University of Alabama, Birmingham, Birmingham, AL, USA. mford@uab.edu

Journal: Arch Phys Med Rehabil. 2010 Aug;91(8):1255-61.

Abstract Link: http://www.medifocus.com/abstracts.php?gid=NR013&ID=20684907

76.

A 12-year population-based study of psychosis in Parkinson disease.

Authors: Forsaa EB; Larsen JP; Wentzel-Larsen T; Goetz CG; Stebbins GT; Aarsland D; Alves G

Institution: The Norwegian Centre for Movement Disorders, Stavanger University Hospital, Box 8100, N-4068 Stavanger, Norway.

Journal: Arch Neurol. 2010 Aug;67(8):996-1001.

Abstract Link: http://www.medifocus.com/abstracts.php?gid=NR013&ID=20697051

Go to http://www.medifocus.com/links/NR013/0112 for direct online access to the above Abstract Links.

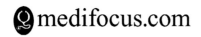

77.

What predicts mortality in Parkinson disease?: a prospective population-based long-term study.

Authors:	Forsaa EB; Larsen JP; Wentzel-Larsen T; Alves G
Institution:	The Norwegian Center for Movement Disorders, Stavanger University Hospital, Box 8100, N-4068 Stavanger, Norway. foeb@sus.no
Journal:	Neurology. 2010 Oct 5;75(14):1270-6.
Abstract Link:	http://www.medifocus.com/abstracts.php?gid=NR013&ID=20921512

78.

Prenatal and early life factors and risk of Parkinson's disease.

Authors:	Gardener H; Gao X; Chen H; Schwarzschild MA; Spiegelman D; Ascherio A
Institution:	Department of Epidemiology, Harvard School of Public Health, Boston, Massachusetts, USA. hgardener@med.miami.edu
Journal:	Mov Disord. 2010 Aug 15;25(11):1560-7.
Abstract Link:	http://www.medifocus.com/abstracts.php?gid=NR013&ID=20740569

79.

The estimated life expectancy in a community cohort of Parkinson's disease patients with and without dementia, compared with the UK population.

Authors:	Hobson P; Meara J; Ishihara-Paul L
Institution:	Academic Unit (North Wales), Cardiff University, Glan Clwyd Hospital, Rhyl, UK. peterhobson@hotmail.com
Journal:	J Neurol Neurosurg Psychiatry. 2010 Oct;81(10):1093-8. Epub 2010 Jun 22.
Abstract Link:	http://www.medifocus.com/abstracts.php?gid=NR013&ID=20571039

Go to http://www.medifocus.com/links/NR013/0112 for direct online access to the above Abstract Links.

@medifocus.com

80.

Depression and major depressive disorder in patients with Parkinson's disease.

Authors:	Inoue T; Kitagawa M; Tanaka T; Nakagawa S; Koyama T
Institution:	Department of Psychiatry, Hokkaido University Graduate School of Medicine, Kita-ku, Sapporo 060-8638, Japan. tinoue@med.hokudai.ac.jp
Journal:	Mov Disord. 2010 Jan 15;25(1):44-9.
Abstract Link:	http://www.medifocus.com/abstracts.php?gid=NR013&ID=20014057

81.

Multi-modal hallucinations and cognitive function in Parkinson's disease.

Authors:	Katzen H; Myerson C; Papapetropoulos S; Nahab F; Gallo B; Levin B
Institution:	Division of Neuropsychology, Department of Neurology, University of Miami, Miller School of Medicine, Miami, FL 33136, USA. hkatzen@med.miami.edu
Journal:	Dement Geriatr Cogn Disord. 2010;30(1):51-6. Epub 2010 Jul 31.
Abstract Link:	http://www.medifocus.com/abstracts.php?gid=NR013&ID=20689283

82.

Compulsive behaviors in patients with Parkinson's disease.

Authors:	Kenangil G; Ozekmekci S; Sohtaoglu M; Erginoz E
Institution:	Department of Neurology, Sisli Etfal Education and Research Hospital, Istanbul, Turkey.
Journal:	Neurologist. 2010 May;16(3):192-5.
Abstract Link:	http://www.medifocus.com/abstracts.php?gid=NR013&ID=20445429

Go to http://www.medifocus.com/links/NR013/0112 for direct online access to the above Abstract Links.

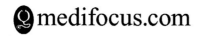

83.

Predictors of future falls in Parkinson disease.

Authors:	Kerr GK; Worringham CJ; Cole MH; Lacherez PF; Wood JM; Silburn PA
Institution:	School of Human Movement Studies, Institute of Health and Biomedical Innovation, Royal Brisbane and Women's Hospital, Queensland, Australia. g.kerr@qut.edu.au
Journal:	Neurology. 2010 Jul 13;75(2):116-24. Epub 2010 Jun 23.
Abstract Link:	http://www.medifocus.com/abstracts.php?gid=NR013&ID=20574039

84.

Talking while walking: Cognitive loading and injurious falls in Parkinson's disease.

Authors:	LaPointe LL; Stierwalt JA; Maitland CG
Institution:	Florida State University, Tallahassee, FL, USA. lllapointe@fsu.edu
Journal:	Int J Speech Lang Pathol. 2010 Oct;12(5):455-9.
Abstract Link:	http://www.medifocus.com/abstracts.php?gid=NR013&ID=20632845

85.

The impact of and the factors associated with drooling in Parkinson's disease.

Authors:	Leibner J; Ramjit A; Sedig L; Dai Y; Wu SS; Jacobson C 4th; Okun MS; Rodriguez RL; Malaty IA; Fernandez HH
Institution:	College of Medicine, University of Florida, Gainesville, FL 32610, USA.
Journal:	Parkinsonism Relat Disord. 2010 Aug;16(7):475-7. Epub 2010 Jan 12.
Abstract Link:	http://www.medifocus.com/abstracts.php?gid=NR013&ID=20064737

Go to http://www.medifocus.com/links/NR013/0112 for direct online access to the above Abstract Links.

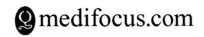
86.

Frequency, type and factors associated with the use of complementary and alternative medicine in patients with Parkinson's disease at a neurological outpatient clinic.

Authors: Lokk J; Nilsson M
Institution: Institution of Neurobiology, Care Sciences and Society, Karolinska Institutet, Geriatric Dept, Karolinska University Hospital Huddinge, SE-14186 Stockholm, Sweden. johan.lokk@karolinska.se
Journal: Parkinsonism Relat Disord. 2010 Sep;16(8):540-4. Epub 2010 Jul 23.
Abstract Link: http://www.medifocus.com/abstracts.php?gid=NR013&ID=20655794

87.

Deciding to institutionalize: why do family members cease caregiving at home?

Authors: McLennon SM; Habermann B; Davis LL
Institution: School of Nursing, Indiana University, Indianapolis, IN, USA. smclenno@iupui.edu
Journal: J Neurosci Nurs. 2010 Apr;42(2):95-103.
Abstract Link: http://www.medifocus.com/abstracts.php?gid=NR013&ID=20422795

88.

Dietary intake of folate, vitamin B6, vitamin B12 and riboflavin and risk of Parkinson's disease: a case-control study in Japan.

Authors: Murakami K; Miyake Y; Sasaki S; Tanaka K; Fukushima W; Kiyohara C; Tsuboi Y; Yamada T; Oeda T; Miki T; Kawamura N; Sakae N; Fukuyama H; Hirota Y; Nagai M
Institution: Department of Social and Preventive Epidemiology, School of Public Health, University of Tokyo, Hongo 7-3-1, Bunkyo-ku, Tokyo 113-0033, Japan. kenmrkm@m.u-tokyo.ac.jp
Journal: Br J Nutr. 2010 Sep;104(5):757-64. Epub 2010 Mar 26.
Abstract Link: http://www.medifocus.com/abstracts.php?gid=NR013&ID=20338075

Go to http://www.medifocus.com/links/NR013/0112 for direct online access to the above Abstract Links.

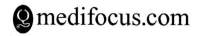

89.

The cause of death in idiopathic Parkinson's disease.

Authors: Pennington S; Snell K; Lee M; Walker R

Institution: ST3 Palliative Medicine Marie Curie hospice, Marie Curie Drive, Newcastle upon Tyne, UK.

Journal: Parkinsonism Relat Disord. 2010 Aug;16(7):434-7. Epub 2010 May 31.

Abstract Link: http://www.medifocus.com/abstracts.php?gid=NR013&ID=20570207

90.

Parkinson's disease symptoms: the patient's perspective.

Authors: Politis M; Wu K; Molloy S; G Bain P; Chaudhuri KR; Piccini P

Institution: Department of Clinical Neurosciences, Faculty of Medicine, Hammersmith Hospital, Imperial College, London, United Kingdom. marios.politis@imperial.ac.uk

Journal: Mov Disord. 2010 Aug 15;25(11):1646-51.

Abstract Link: http://www.medifocus.com/abstracts.php?gid=NR013&ID=20629164

91.

Major life events and risk of Parkinson's disease.

Authors: Rod NH; Hansen J; Schernhammer E; Ritz B

Institution: Institute of Public Health, University of Copenhagen, Department of Social Medicine, Copenhagen, Denmark. n.rod@pubhealth.ku.dk

Journal: Mov Disord. 2010 Aug 15;25(11):1639-45.

Abstract Link: http://www.medifocus.com/abstracts.php?gid=NR013&ID=20602449

Go to http://www.medifocus.com/links/NR013/0112 for direct online access to the above Abstract Links.

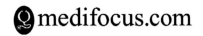

92.

Environmental and familial risk factors of Parkinsons disease: case-control study.

Authors: Sanyal J; Chakraborty DP; Sarkar B; Banerjee TK; Mukherjee SC; Ray BC; Rao VR

Institution: Anthropological Survey of India, Jawaharlal Nehru Road, India.

Journal: Can J Neurol Sci. 2010 Sep;37(5):637-42.

Abstract Link: http://www.medifocus.com/abstracts.php?gid=NR013&ID=21059511

93.

Predictors of cognitive outcomes in early Parkinson disease patients: The National Institutes of Health Exploratory Trials in Parkinson Disease (NET-PD) experience.

Authors: Schneider JS; Elm JJ; Parashos SA; Ravina BM; Galpern WR

Institution: Department of Pathology, Anatomy and Cell Biology, Thomas Jefferson University, 1020 Locust Street, 521 JAH, Philadelphia, PA 19107, USA. jay.schneider@jefferson.edu

Journal: Parkinsonism Relat Disord. 2010 Sep;16(8):507-12. Epub 2010 Jul 2.

Abstract Link: http://www.medifocus.com/abstracts.php?gid=NR013&ID=20598621

94.

Gum chewing improves swallow frequency and latency in Parkinson patients: a preliminary study.

Authors: South AR; Somers SM; Jog MS

Institution: cMovement Disorders Clinic, London Health Sciences Centre, 339 Windemere Blvd, A 10-026, London, Ontario Canada. asouth4@uwo.ca

Journal: Neurology. 2010 Apr 13;74(15):1198-202.

Abstract Link: http://www.medifocus.com/abstracts.php?gid=NR013&ID=20385891

Go to http://www.medifocus.com/links/NR013/0112 for direct online access to the above Abstract Links.

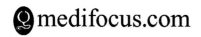

95.

Parkinson disease: sialorrhea and Parkinson disease--novel treatment approaches.

Authors: Troche MS; Fernandez HH
Journal: Nat Rev Neurol. 2010 Aug;6(8):423-4.
Abstract Link: http://www.medifocus.com/abstracts.php?gid=NR013&ID=20689564

96.

Marked improvement of psychotic symptoms after electroconvulsive therapy in Parkinson disease.

Authors: Ueda S; Koyama K; Okubo Y
Institution: Department of Neuropsychiatry, Nippon Medical School, Tokyo, Japan. sat333@nms.ac.jp
Journal: J ECT. 2010 Jun;26(2):111-5.
Abstract Link: http://www.medifocus.com/abstracts.php?gid=NR013&ID=20386461

97.

Physical activities and future risk of Parkinson disease.

Authors: Xu Q; Park Y; Huang X; Hollenbeck A; Blair A; Schatzkin A; Chen H
Institution: Epidemiology Branch, National Institute of Environmental Health Sciences, 111 T.W. Alexander Drive, Research Triangle Park, NC 27709, USA.
Journal: Neurology. 2010 Jul 27;75(4):341-8.
Abstract Link: http://www.medifocus.com/abstracts.php?gid=NR013&ID=20660864

Go to http://www.medifocus.com/links/NR013/0112 for direct online access to the above Abstract Links.

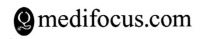

98.

Practice Parameter: treatment of nonmotor symptoms of Parkinson disease: report of the Quality Standards Subcommittee of the American Academy of Neurology.

Authors:	Zesiewicz TA; Sullivan KL; Arnulf I; Chaudhuri KR; Morgan JC; Gronseth GS; Miyasaki J; Iverson DJ; Weiner WJ
Institution:	University of South Florida, Tampa, USA.
Journal:	Neurology. 2010 Mar 16;74(11):924-31.
Abstract Link:	http://www.medifocus.com/abstracts.php?gid=NR013&ID=20231670

99.

Pathologic findings in retinal pigment epithelial cell implantation for Parkinson disease.

Authors:	Farag ES; Vinters HV; Bronstein J
Institution:	Movement Disorders Program, UCLA Department of Neurology, 300 UCLA Medical Plaza Ste. B200, Los Angeles, CA 90095, USA. efarag@mednet.ucla.edu
Journal:	Neurology. 2009 Oct 6;73(14):1095-102. Epub 2009 Sep 2.
Abstract Link:	http://www.medifocus.com/abstracts.php?gid=NR013&ID=19726750

100.

Family history of melanoma and Parkinson disease risk.

Authors:	Gao X; Simon KC; Han J; Schwarzschild MA; Ascherio A
Institution:	Channing Laboratory, Department of Medicine, Brigham and Women's Hospital and Harvard Medical School, Boston, MA 02115, USA. xiang.gao@channing.harvard.edu
Journal:	Neurology. 2009 Oct 20;73(16):1286-91.
Abstract Link:	http://www.medifocus.com/abstracts.php?gid=NR013&ID=19841380

Go to http://www.medifocus.com/links/NR013/0112 for direct online access to the above Abstract Links.

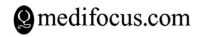

101.

Botulinum toxin A for overactive bladder and detrusor muscle overactivity in patients with Parkinson's disease and multiple system atrophy.

Authors:	Giannantoni A; Rossi A; Mearini E; Del Zingaro M; Porena M; Berardelli A
Institution:	Department of Urology and Andrology, Ospedale Santa Maria della Misericordia, University of Perugia, Perugia, Italy. agianton@libero.it
Journal:	J Urol. 2009 Oct;182(4):1453-7. Epub 2009 Aug 15.
Abstract Link:	http://www.medifocus.com/abstracts.php?gid=NR013&ID=19683298

102.

Jean-Martin Charcot and his vibratory chair for Parkinson disease.

Author:	Goetz CG
Institution:	Department of Neurological Sciences, Rush University Medical Center, Chicago, IL, USA. cgoetz@rush.edu
Journal:	Neurology. 2009 Aug 11;73(6):475-8.
Abstract Link:	http://www.medifocus.com/abstracts.php?gid=NR013&ID=19667323

103.

Inner retinal layer thinning in Parkinson disease.

Authors:	Hajee ME; March WF; Lazzaro DR; Wolintz AH; Shrier EM; Glazman S; Bodis-Wollner IG
Institution:	Department of Neurology, State University of New York Downstate Medical Center, Brooklyn, NY 11203, USA.
Journal:	Arch Ophthalmol. 2009 Jun;127(6):737-41.
Abstract Link:	http://www.medifocus.com/abstracts.php?gid=NR013&ID=19506190

Go to http://www.medifocus.com/links/NR013/0112 for direct online access to the above Abstract Links.

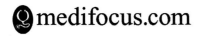

104.

Cerebellar magnetic stimulation decreases levodopa-induced dyskinesias in Parkinson disease.

Authors: Koch G; Brusa L; Carrillo F; Lo Gerfo E; Torriero S; Oliveri M; Mir P; Caltagirone C; Stanzione P
Institution: Laboratorio di Neurologia Clinica e Comportamentale Fondazione Santa Lucia, IRCCS Via Ardeatina 306 00179 Roma, Italy. g.koch@hsantalucia.it
Journal: Neurology. 2009 Jul 14;73(2):113-9.
Abstract Link: http://www.medifocus.com/abstracts.php?gid=NR013&ID=19597133

105.

Clinical features in early Parkinson disease and survival.

Authors: Lo RY; Tanner CM; Albers KB; Leimpeter AD; Fross RD; Bernstein AL; McGuire V; Quesenberry CP; Nelson LM; Van Den Eeden SK
Institution: The Parkinson's Institute and Clinical Center, Sunnyvale, CA 94085, USA.
Journal: Arch Neurol. 2009 Nov;66(11):1353-8.
Abstract Link: http://www.medifocus.com/abstracts.php?gid=NR013&ID=19901166

106.

Quality of life in relation to mood, coping strategies, and dyskinesia in Parkinson's disease.

Authors: Montel S; Bonnet AM; Bungener C
Institution: Laboratory of Clinical Psychopathology and Neuropsychology, University of Paris Descartes, Boulogne Billancourt Paris, France. montel.sebastien@wanadoo.fr
Journal: J Geriatr Psychiatry Neurol. 2009 Jun;22(2):95-102. Epub 2009 Jan 15.
Abstract Link: http://www.medifocus.com/abstracts.php?gid=NR013&ID=19150974

Go to http://www.medifocus.com/links/NR013/0112 for direct online access to the above Abstract Links.

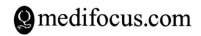

107.

Course in Parkinson disease subtypes: A 39-year clinicopathologic study.

Authors: Rajput AH; Voll A; Rajput ML; Robinson CA; Rajput A

Institution: Division of Neurology, Department of Pathology, Saskatoon Health Region/University of Saskatchewan, Canada.

Journal: Neurology. 2009 Jul 21;73(3):206-12.

Abstract Link: http://www.medifocus.com/abstracts.php?gid=NR013&ID=19620608

108.

Elevated serum pesticide levels and risk of Parkinson disease.

Authors: Richardson JR; Shalat SL; Buckley B; Winnik B; O'Suilleabhain P; Diaz-Arrastia R; Reisch J; German DC

Institution: Robert Wood Johnson Medical School, Piscataway, New Jersey, USA. jricha3@eohsi.rutgers.edu

Journal: Arch Neurol. 2009 Jul;66(7):870-5.

Abstract Link: http://www.medifocus.com/abstracts.php?gid=NR013&ID=19597089

109.

Autoimmune disease and risk for Parkinson disease: a population-based case-control study.

Authors: Rugbjerg K; Friis S; Ritz B; Schernhammer ES; Korbo L; Olsen JH

Institution: Institute of Cancer Epidemiology, Danish Cancer Society, Strandboulevarden 49, DK-2100 Copenhagen, Denmark. rugbjerg@cancer.dk

Journal: Neurology. 2009 Nov 3;73(18):1462-8. Epub 2009 Sep 23.

Abstract Link: http://www.medifocus.com/abstracts.php?gid=NR013&ID=19776374

Go to http://www.medifocus.com/links/NR013/0112 for direct online access to the above Abstract Links.

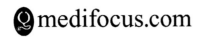

110.

Anemia or low hemoglobin levels preceding Parkinson disease: a case-control study.

Authors:	Savica R; Grossardt BR; Carlin JM; Icen M; Bower JH; Ahlskog JE; Maraganore DM; Steensma DP; Rocca WA
Institution:	Department of Neurology, College of Medicine, Mayo Clinic, Rochester, MN 55905, USA. rocca@mayo.edu
Journal:	Neurology. 2009 Oct 27;73(17):1381-7.
Abstract Link:	http://www.medifocus.com/abstracts.php?gid=NR013&ID=19858460

111.

Medical records documentation of constipation preceding Parkinson disease: A case-control study.

Authors:	Savica R; Carlin JM; Grossardt BR; Bower JH; Ahlskog JE; Maraganore DM; Bharucha AE; Rocca WA
Institution:	Department of Neurology, Mayo Clinic, Rochester, MN 55905, USA.
Journal:	Neurology. 2009 Nov 24;73(21):1752-8.
Abstract Link:	http://www.medifocus.com/abstracts.php?gid=NR013&ID=19933976

112.

Gait analysis in patients with Parkinson's disease off dopaminergic therapy.

Authors:	Svehlik M; Zwick EB; Steinwender G; Linhart WE; Schwingenschuh P; Katschnig P; Ott E; Enzinger C
Institution:	Paediatric Orthopaedic Unit, Department of Paediatric Surgery, Medical University of Graz, Auenbruggerplatz 34, Graz, A-8036, Austria. martin.spejlik@seznam.cz
Journal:	Arch Phys Med Rehabil. 2009 Nov;90(11):1880-6.
Abstract Link:	http://www.medifocus.com/abstracts.php?gid=NR013&ID=19887212

Go to http://www.medifocus.com/links/NR013/0112 for direct online access to the above Abstract Links.

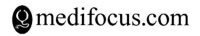

113.

Driving under low-contrast visibility conditions in Parkinson disease.

Authors: Uc EY; Rizzo M; Anderson SW; Dastrup E; Sparks JD; Dawson JD
Institution: Department of Neurology, University of Iowa, Carver College of Medicine, 200 Hawkins Dr., 2RCP, Iowa City, IA 52242, USA. ergun-uc@uiowa.edu
Journal: Neurology. 2009 Oct 6;73(14):1103-10.
Abstract Link: http://www.medifocus.com/abstracts.php?gid=NR013&ID=19805726

114.

Incidence of and risk factors for cognitive impairment in an early Parkinson disease clinical trial cohort.

Authors: Uc EY; McDermott MP; Marder KS; Anderson SW; Litvan I; Como PG; Auinger P; Chou KL; Growdon JC
Institution: Department of Neurology, University of Iowa, Carver College of Medicine, 200 Hawkins Drive-2RCP, Iowa City, IA 52242, USA. ergun-uc@uiowa.edu
Journal: Neurology. 2009 Nov 3;73(18):1469-77.
Abstract Link: http://www.medifocus.com/abstracts.php?gid=NR013&ID=19884574

115.

Road safety in drivers with Parkinson disease.

Authors: Uc EY; Rizzo M; Johnson AM; Dastrup E; Anderson SW; Dawson JD
Institution: Department of Neurology, University of Iowa, Carver College of Medicine, 200 Hawkins Drive-2RCP, Iowa City, IA 52242, USA. ergun-uc@uiowa.edu
Journal: Neurology. 2009 Dec 15;73(24):2112-9.
Abstract Link: http://www.medifocus.com/abstracts.php?gid=NR013&ID=20018639

Go to http://www.medifocus.com/links/NR013/0112 for direct online access to the above Abstract Links.

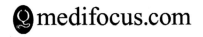 medifocus.com

The distinct cognitive syndromes of Parkinson's disease: 5 year follow-up of the CamPaIGN cohort.

Authors: Williams-Gray CH; Evans JR; Goris A; Foltynie T; Ban M; Robbins TW; Brayne C; Kolachana BS; Weinberger DR; Sawcer SJ; Barker RA

Institution: Cambridge Centre for Brain Repair, Department of Clinical Neurosciences, University of Cambridge, Forvie Site, Robinson Way, Cambridge, CB2 0PY, UK. chm27@cam.ac.uk

Journal: Brain. 2009 Nov;132(Pt 11):2958-69. Epub 2009 Oct 7.

Abstract Link: http://www.medifocus.com/abstracts.php?gid=NR013&ID=19812213

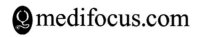

Drug Therapy Articles

117.

Patterns and trends in antipsychotic prescribing for Parkinson disease psychosis.

Authors: Weintraub D; Chen P; Ignacio RV; Mamikonyan E; Kales HC

Institution: Department of Psychiatry, University of Pennsylvania, Philadelphia, PA 19104, USA. daniel.weintraub@uphs.upenn.edu

Journal: Arch Neurol. 2011 Jul;68(7):899-904.

Abstract Link: http://www.medifocus.com/abstracts.php?gid=NR013&ID=21747029

118.

Zonisamide: a new drug for Parkinson's disease.

Author: Murata M

Institution: Department of Neurology, National Center Hospital, National Center of Neurology and Psychiatry, Kodaira, Tokyo, Japan. mihom@ncnp.go.jp

Journal: Drugs Today (Barc). 2010 Apr;46(4):251-8.

Abstract Link: http://www.medifocus.com/abstracts.php?gid=NR013&ID=20502722

119.

Current use of clozapine in Parkinson disease and related disorders.

Authors: Thomas AA; Friedman JH

Institution: Alpert Medical School, Brown University, Providence, RI 02886, USA.

Journal: Clin Neuropharmacol. 2010 Jan-Feb;33(1):14-6.

Abstract Link: http://www.medifocus.com/abstracts.php?gid=NR013&ID=20023573

Go to http://www.medifocus.com/links/NR013/0112 for direct online access to the above Abstract Links.

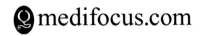

Clinical Trials Articles

120.

Intermittent theta-burst transcranial magnetic stimulation for treatment of Parkinson disease.

Authors:	Benninger DH; Berman BD; Houdayer E; Pal N; Luckenbaugh DA; Schneider L; Miranda S; Hallett M
Institution:	Department of Neurology, University Hospital of Basel, Petersgraben 4, 4051 Basel, Switzerland. benningerd@uhbs.ch
Journal:	Neurology. 2011 Feb 15;76(7):601-9.
Abstract Link:	http://www.medifocus.com/abstracts.php?gid=NR013&ID=21321333

121.

Cognitive-behavioral therapy for depression in Parkinson's disease: a randomized, controlled trial.

Authors:	Dobkin RD; Menza M; Allen LA; Gara MA; Mark MH; Tiu J; Bienfait KL; Friedman J
Institution:	Department of Psychiatry, University of Medicine and Dentistry of New Jersey-Robert Wood Johnson Medical School, Piscataway, USA. dobkinro@umdnj.edu
Journal:	Am J Psychiatry. 2011 Oct;168(10):1066-74. Epub 2011 Jun 15.
Abstract Link:	http://www.medifocus.com/abstracts.php?gid=NR013&ID=21676990

122.

Methylphenidate for gait impairment in Parkinson disease: a randomized clinical trial.

Authors:	Espay AJ; Dwivedi AK; Payne M; Gaines L; Vaughan JE; Maddux BN; Slevin JT; Gartner M; Sahay A; Revilla FJ; Duker AP; Shukla R
Institution:	Department of Neurology, University of Cincinnati, Cincinnati, OH 45267-0525, USA. alberto.espay@uc.edu
Journal:	Neurology. 2011 Apr 5;76(14):1256-62.
Abstract Link:	http://www.medifocus.com/abstracts.php?gid=NR013&ID=21464430

Go to http://www.medifocus.com/links/NR013/0112 for direct online access to the above Abstract Links.

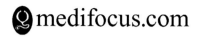

123.

High prevalence of hypovitaminosis D status in patients with early Parkinson disease.

Authors: Evatt ML; DeLong MR; Kumari M; Auinger P; McDermott MP; Tangpricha V

Institution: Department of Neurology, Emory University School of Medicine, 1841 Clifton Rd NE, Atlanta, GA 30329, USA. mevatt@emory.edu

Journal: Arch Neurol. 2011 Mar;68(3):314-9.

Abstract Link: http://www.medifocus.com/abstracts.php?gid=NR013&ID=21403017

124.

Modified constraint-induced movement therapy improves fine and gross motor performance of the upper limb in Parkinson disease.

Authors: Lee KS; Lee WH; Hwang S

Institution: Department of Physical Therapy, College of Health Science and Social Welfare, Sahmyook University, Seoul, Korea.

Journal: Am J Phys Med Rehabil. 2011 May;90(5):380-6.

Abstract Link: http://www.medifocus.com/abstracts.php?gid=NR013&ID=21389845

125.

Parkinson's disease progression at 30 years: a study of subthalamic deep brain-stimulated patients.

Authors: Merola A; Zibetti M; Angrisano S; Rizzi L; Ricchi V; Artusi CA; Lanotte M; Rizzone MG; Lopiano L

Institution: Department of Neuroscience, University of Torino, Via Cherasco 15, 10126 Turin, Italy. aristidemerola@hotmail.com

Journal: Brain. 2011 Jul;134(Pt 7):2074-84. Epub 2011 Jun 11.

Abstract Link: http://www.medifocus.com/abstracts.php?gid=NR013&ID=21666262

Go to http://www.medifocus.com/links/NR013/0112 for direct online access to the above Abstract Links.

126.

Virtual reality for gait training: can it induce motor learning to enhance complex walking and reduce fall risk in patients with Parkinson's disease?

Authors: Mirelman A; Maidan I; Herman T; Deutsch JE; Giladi N; Hausdorff JM

Institution: Movement Disorders Unit, Department of Neurology, Tel Aviv Sourasky Medical Center, Israel. anatmi@tasmc.health.gov.il

Journal: J Gerontol A Biol Sci Med Sci. 2011 Feb;66(2):234-40. Epub 2010 Nov 24.

Abstract Link: http://www.medifocus.com/abstracts.php?gid=NR013&ID=21106702

127.

Excessive daytime sleepiness in multiple system atrophy (SLEEMSA study).

Authors: Moreno-Lopez C; Santamaria J; Salamero M; Del Sorbo F; Albanese A; Pellecchia MT; Barone P; Overeem S; Bloem B; Aarden W; Canesi M; Antonini A; Duerr S; Wenning GK; Poewe W; Rubino A; Meco G; Schneider SA; Bhatia KP; Djaldetti R; Coelho M; Sampaio C; Cochen V; Hellriegel H; Deuschl G; Colosimo C; Marsili L; Gasser T; Tolosa E

Institution: Movement Disorders Unit, Department of Neurology, Hospital Clinic of Barcelona, University of Barcelona Medical School and Centro de Investigacion Biomedica en Red sobre Enfermedades Neurodegenerativas, 08036 Barcelona, Spain.

Journal: Arch Neurol. 2011 Feb;68(2):223-30.

Abstract Link: http://www.medifocus.com/abstracts.php?gid=NR013&ID=21320989

Go to http://www.medifocus.com/links/NR013/0112 for direct online access to the above Abstract Links.

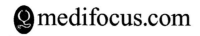

128.

Unilateral subdural motor cortex stimulation improves essential tremor but not Parkinson's disease.

Authors:	Moro E; Schwalb JM; Piboolnurak P; Poon YY; Hamani C; Hung SW; Arenovich T; Lang AE; Chen R; Lozano AM
Institution:	Movement Disorders Centre, Division of Neurology, Department of Medicine, University of Toronto, Toronto Western Hospital, University Health Network,Toronto, ON M5T2S8, Canada. elena.moro@uhn.on.ca
Journal:	Brain. 2011 Jul;134(Pt 7):2096-105. Epub 2011 Jun 6.
Abstract Link:	http://www.medifocus.com/abstracts.php?gid=NR013&ID=21646329

129.

Extended-release pramipexole in early Parkinson disease: a 33-week randomized controlled trial.

Authors:	Poewe W; Rascol O; Barone P; Hauser RA; Mizuno Y; Haaksma M; Salin L; Juhel N; Schapira AH
Institution:	Innsbruck Medical University, Innsbruck, Austria. werner.poewe@i-med.ac.at
Journal:	Neurology. 2011 Aug 23;77(8):759-66. Epub 2011 Aug 10.
Abstract Link:	http://www.medifocus.com/abstracts.php?gid=NR013&ID=21832218

130.

Extended-release pramipexole in advanced Parkinson disease: a randomized controlled trial.

Authors:	Schapira AH; Barone P; Hauser RA; Mizuno Y; Rascol O; Busse M; Salin L; Juhel N; Poewe W
Institution:	Institute of Neurology, University College London, London, UK. a.schapira@ucl.ac.uk
Journal:	Neurology. 2011 Aug 23;77(8):767-74. Epub 2011 Aug 10.
Abstract Link:	http://www.medifocus.com/abstracts.php?gid=NR013&ID=21832216

Go to http://www.medifocus.com/links/NR013/0112 for direct online access to the above Abstract Links.

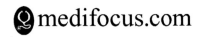

131.

Aquatic therapy versus conventional land-based therapy for Parkinson's disease: an open-label pilot study.

Authors: Vivas J; Arias P; Cudeiro J

Institution: Neuroscience and Motor Control Group (NEUROcom), Department of Physical Therapy, University of A Coruna, A Coruna, Spain.

Journal: Arch Phys Med Rehabil. 2011 Aug;92(8):1202-10.

Abstract Link: http://www.medifocus.com/abstracts.php?gid=NR013&ID=21807139

132.

Dopamine agonists and risk: impulse control disorders in Parkinson's disease.

Authors: Voon V; Gao J; Brezing C; Symmonds M; Ekanayake V; Fernandez H; Dolan RJ; Hallett M

Institution: Behavioural and Clinical Neurosciences Institute, Department of Experimental Psychology, Downing Site, University of Cambridge, Cambridge CB2 3EB, UK. vv247@cam.ac.uk

Journal: Brain. 2011 May;134(Pt 5):1438-46.

Abstract Link: http://www.medifocus.com/abstracts.php?gid=NR013&ID=21596771

133.

Mild cognitive impairment in Parkinson disease: a multicenter pooled analysis.

Authors: Aarsland D; Bronnick K; Williams-Gray C; Weintraub D; Marder K; Kulisevsky J; Burn D; Barone P; Pagonabarraga J; Allcock L; Santangelo G; Foltynie T; Janvin C; Larsen JP; Barker RA; Emre M

Institution: Stavanger University Hospital, Psychiatric Division, PO Box 8100, 4068 Stavanger, Norway. daarsland@gmail.com

Journal: Neurology. 2010 Sep 21;75(12):1062-9.

Abstract Link: http://www.medifocus.com/abstracts.php?gid=NR013&ID=20855849

Go to http://www.medifocus.com/links/NR013/0112 for direct online access to the above Abstract Links.

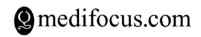
134.

Controlled trial on the effect of 10 days low-frequency repetitive transcranial magnetic stimulation (rTMS) on motor signs in Parkinson's disease.

Authors: Arias P; Vivas J; Grieve KL; Cudeiro J
Institution: Neuroscience and Motor Control Group (NEUROcom), Department of Medicine-INEF and Institute for Biomedical Research (INIBIC), University of A Coruna, Spain.
Journal: Mov Disord. 2010 Sep 15;25(12):1830-8.
Abstract Link: http://www.medifocus.com/abstracts.php?gid=NR013&ID=20669300

135.

Double-blind, randomized, placebo controlled trial on the effect of 10 days low-frequency rTMS over the vertex on sleep in Parkinson's disease.

Authors: Arias P; Vivas J; Grieve KL; Cudeiro J
Institution: Neuroscience and Motor Control Group (NEUROcom), Department of Medicine-INEF and Institute for Biomedical Research (INIBIC), University of A Coruna, Spain.
Journal: Sleep Med. 2010 Sep;11(8):759-65. Epub 2010 Jul 31.
Abstract Link: http://www.medifocus.com/abstracts.php?gid=NR013&ID=20674489

136.

Transcranial direct current stimulation for the treatment of Parkinson's disease.

Authors: Benninger DH; Lomarev M; Lopez G; Wassermann EM; Li X; Considine E; Hallett M
Institution: Medical Neurology Branch, National Institute of Neurological Disorders and Stroke, National Institutes of Health, Bethesda, Maryland 20892, USA. benningerd@ninds.nih.gov
Journal: J Neurol Neurosurg Psychiatry. 2010 Oct;81(10):1105-11.
Abstract Link: http://www.medifocus.com/abstracts.php?gid=NR013&ID=20870863

Go to http://www.medifocus.com/links/NR013/0112 for direct online access to the above Abstract Links.

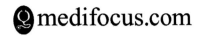

137.

Pramipexole for the treatment of depressive symptoms in patients with Parkinson's disease: a randomised, double-blind, placebo-controlled trial.

Authors: Bxarone P; Poewe W; Albrecht S; Debieuvre C; Massey D; Rascol O; Tolosa E; Weintraub D

Institution: Department of Neurological Sciences, University of Naples Federico II and IDC Hermitage Capodimonte, Naples, Italy. barone@unina.it

Journal: Lancet Neurol. 2010 Jun;9(6):573-80. Epub 2010 May 7.

Abstract Link: http://www.medifocus.com/abstracts.php?gid=NR013&ID=20452823

138.

Effects of a central cholinesterase inhibitor on reducing falls in Parkinson disease.

Authors: Chung KA; Lobb BM; Nutt JG; Horak FB

Institution: Department of Neurology, Oregon Health & Science University, Portland, OR, USA. chungka@ohsu.edu

Journal: Neurology. 2010 Oct 5;75(14):1263-9. Epub 2010 Sep 1.

Abstract Link: http://www.medifocus.com/abstracts.php?gid=NR013&ID=20810998

139.

The MoCA: well-suited screen for cognitive impairment in Parkinson disease.

Authors: Dalrymple-Alford JC; MacAskill MR; Nakas CT; Livingston L; Graham C; Crucian GP; Melzer TR; Kirwan J; Keenan R; Wells S; Porter RJ; Watts R; Anderson TJ

Institution: Van der Veer Institute for Parkinson's and Brain Research, 66 Stewart St., Christchurch 8011, New Zealand. john.dalrymple-alford@canterbury.ac.nz

Journal: Neurology. 2010 Nov 9;75(19):1717-25.

Abstract Link: http://www.medifocus.com/abstracts.php?gid=NR013&ID=21060094

Go to http://www.medifocus.com/links/NR013/0112 for direct online access to the above Abstract Links.

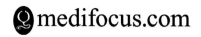
140.

Risk factors for executive dysfunction after subthalamic nucleus stimulation in Parkinson's disease.

Authors:	Daniels C; Krack P; Volkmann J; Pinsker MO; Krause M; Tronnier V; Kloss M; Schnitzler A; Wojtecki L; Botzel K; Danek A; Hilker R; Sturm V; Kupsch A; Karner E; Deuschl G; Witt K
Institution:	Department of Neurology, Christian-Albrechts-University, Kiel, Germany.
Journal:	Mov Disord. 2010 Aug 15;25(11):1583-9.
Abstract Link:	http://www.medifocus.com/abstracts.php?gid=NR013&ID=20589868

141.

The impact of antidepressant treatment on cognitive functioning in depressed patients with Parkinson's disease.

Authors:	Dobkin RD; Menza M; Bienfait KL; Gara M; Marin H; Mark MH; Dicke A; Troster A
Institution:	Department of Psychiatry, UMDNJ, Robert Wood Johnson Medical School, D317, 675 Hoes Lane, Piscataway, NJ 08854, USA. dobkinro@umdnj.edu
Journal:	J Neuropsychiatry Clin Neurosci. 2010 Spring;22(2):188-95.
Abstract Link:	http://www.medifocus.com/abstracts.php?gid=NR013&ID=20463113

142.

Comparing exercise in Parkinson's disease--the Berlin LSVT(R)BIG study.

Authors:	Ebersbach G; Ebersbach A; Edler D; Kaufhold O; Kusch M; Kupsch A; Wissel J
Institution:	Movement Disorders Clinic, Beelitz-Heilstatten, Germany. ebersbach@parkinson-beelitz.de
Journal:	Mov Disord. 2010 Sep 15;25(12):1902-8.
Abstract Link:	http://www.medifocus.com/abstracts.php?gid=NR013&ID=20669294

Go to http://www.medifocus.com/links/NR013/0112 for direct online access to the above Abstract Links.

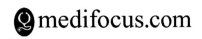

143.

Safety and efficacy of perampanel in advanced Parkinson's disease: a randomized, placebo-controlled study.

Authors: Eggert K; Squillacote D; Barone P; Dodel R; Katzenschlager R; Emre M; Lees AJ; Rascol O; Poewe W; Tolosa E; Trenkwalder C; Onofrj M; Stocchi F; Nappi G; Kostic V; Potic J; Ruzicka E; Oertel W

Institution: German Competence Network on Parkinson's Disease, Department of Neurology, Philipps-University Marburg, Marburg, Germany.

Journal: Mov Disord. 2010 May 15;25(7):896-905.

Abstract Link: http://www.medifocus.com/abstracts.php?gid=NR013&ID=20461807

144.

Memantine for patients with Parkinson's disease dementia or dementia with Lewy bodies: a randomised, double-blind, placebo-controlled trial.

Authors: Emre M; Tsolaki M; Bonuccelli U; Destee A; Tolosa E; Kutzelnigg A; Ceballos-Baumann A; Zdravkovic S; Bladstrom A; Jones R

Institution: Istanbul University, Istanbul Faculty of Medicine, Istanbul, Turkey. muratemre@superonline.com

Journal: Lancet Neurol. 2010 Oct;9(10):969-77. Epub 2010 Aug 20.

Abstract Link: http://www.medifocus.com/abstracts.php?gid=NR013&ID=20729148

145.

Pallidal versus subthalamic deep-brain stimulation for Parkinson's disease.

Authors: Follett KA; Weaver FM; Stern M; Hur K; Harris CL; Luo P; Marks WJ Jr; Rothlind J; Sagher O; Moy C; Pahwa R; Burchiel K; Hogarth P; Lai EC; Duda JE; Holloway K; Samii A; Horn S; Bronstein JM; Stoner G; Starr PA; Simpson R; Baltuch G; De Salles A; Huang GD; Reda DJ

Institution: Iowa City Veterans Affairs Medical Center, Iowa City, USA.

Journal: N Engl J Med. 2010 Jun 3;362(22):2077-91.

Abstract Link: http://www.medifocus.com/abstracts.php?gid=NR013&ID=20519680

Go to http://www.medifocus.com/links/NR013/0112 for direct online access to the above Abstract Links.

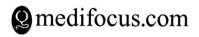

146.

Hallucinations and sleep disorders in PD: ten-year prospective longitudinal study.

Authors: Goetz CG; Ouyang B; Negron A; Stebbins GT
Institution: Movement Disorders Section, Department of Neurological Sciences, Rush University Medical Center, Suite 1106, Chicago, IL 60612, USA. cgoetz@rush.edu
Journal: Neurology. 2010 Nov 16;75(20):1773-9. Epub 2010 Oct 20.
Abstract Link: http://www.medifocus.com/abstracts.php?gid=NR013&ID=20962287

147.

Early treatment benefits of ropinirole prolonged release in Parkinson's disease patients with motor fluctuations.

Authors: Hersh BP; Earl NL; Hauser RA; Stacy M
Institution: Department of Neurology, Harvard Vanguard Medical Associates, Boston, Massachusetts 02215, USA. bonnie_hersh@vmed.org
Journal: Mov Disord. 2010 May 15;25(7):927-31.
Abstract Link: http://www.medifocus.com/abstracts.php?gid=NR013&ID=20461810

148.

Patient perception of dyskinesia in Parkinson's disease.

Authors: Hung SW; Adeli GM; Arenovich T; Fox SH; Lang AE
Institution: Movement Disorders Centre, Toronto Western Hospital and Division of Neurology, University of Toronto, Toronto, Canada.
Journal: J Neurol Neurosurg Psychiatry. 2010 Oct;81(10):1112-5. Epub 2010 Jul 28.
Abstract Link: http://www.medifocus.com/abstracts.php?gid=NR013&ID=20667858

Go to http://www.medifocus.com/links/NR013/0112 for direct online access to the above Abstract Links.

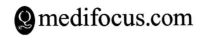

149.

Can reflexology maintain or improve the well-being of people with Parkinson's Disease?

Authors: Johns C; Blake D; Sinclair A

Institution: University of Bedfordshire, Putteridge Bury, Hitchin Road, Luton, LU2 8LE, UK. chris.johns@beds.ac.uk

Journal: Complement Ther Clin Pract. 2010 May;16(2):96-100. Epub 2009 Nov 4.

Abstract Link: http://www.medifocus.com/abstracts.php?gid=NR013&ID=20347841

150.

Use of botulinim toxin-A for the treatment of overactive bladder symptoms in patients with Parkinsons's disease.

Authors: Kulaksizoglu H; Parman Y

Institution: Selcuk University, Selcuklu Medical School, Department of Urology, Turkey. kulaksizoglu@superonline.com

Journal: Parkinsonism Relat Disord. 2010 Sep;16(8):531-4. Epub 2010 Jul 15.

Abstract Link: http://www.medifocus.com/abstracts.php?gid=NR013&ID=20637678

151.

Dopamine cell implantation in Parkinson's disease: long-term clinical and (18)F-FDOPA PET outcomes.

Authors: Ma Y; Tang C; Chaly T; Greene P; Breeze R; Fahn S; Freed C; Dhawan V; Eidelberg D

Institution: Center for Neurosciences, The Feinstein Institute for Medical Research, Manhasset, New York 11030, USA. yma@nshs.edu

Journal: J Nucl Med. 2010 Jan;51(1):7-15. Epub 2009 Dec 15.

Abstract Link: http://www.medifocus.com/abstracts.php?gid=NR013&ID=20008998

Go to http://www.medifocus.com/links/NR013/0112 for direct online access to the above Abstract Links.

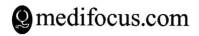

152.

Gene delivery of AAV2-neurturin for Parkinson's disease: a double-blind, randomised, controlled trial.

Authors:	Marks WJ Jr; Bartus RT; Siffert J; Davis CS; Lozano A; Boulis N; Vitek J; Stacy M; Turner D; Verhagen L; Bakay R; Watts R; Guthrie B; Jankovic J; Simpson R; Tagliati M; Alterman R; Stern M; Baltuch G; Starr PA; Larson PS; Ostrem JL; Nutt J; Kieburtz K; Kordower JH; Olanow CW
Institution:	Department of Neurology, University of California San Francisco, San Francisco, CA, USA.
Journal:	Lancet Neurol. 2010 Dec;9(12):1164-72. Epub 2010 Oct 20.
Abstract Link:	http://www.medifocus.com/abstracts.php?gid=NR013&ID=20970382

153.

Treatment of insomnia in Parkinson's disease: a controlled trial of eszopiclone and placebo.

Authors:	Menza M; Dobkin RD; Marin H; Gara M; Bienfait K; Dicke A; Comella CL; Cantor C; Hyer L
Institution:	Department of Psychiatry, Robert Wood Johnson Medical School, Piscataway, New Jersey 08854, USA. menza@umdnj.edu
Journal:	Mov Disord. 2010 Aug 15;25(11):1708-14.
Abstract Link:	http://www.medifocus.com/abstracts.php?gid=NR013&ID=20589875

154.

Clinical efficacy of istradefylline (KW-6002) in Parkinson's disease: a randomized, controlled study.

Authors:	Mizuno Y; Hasegawa K; Kondo T; Kuno S; Yamamoto M
Institution:	Department of Neurology, Research Institute for Diseases of Old Age, Juntendo University School of Medicine, Tokyo, Japan. y_mizuno@juntendo.ac.jp
Journal:	Mov Disord. 2010 Jul 30;25(10):1437-43.
Abstract Link:	http://www.medifocus.com/abstracts.php?gid=NR013&ID=20629136

Go to http://www.medifocus.com/links/NR013/0112 for direct online access to the above Abstract Links.

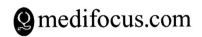

155.

Long-term results of a multicenter study on subthalamic and pallidal stimulation in Parkinson's disease.

Authors:	Moro E; Lozano AM; Pollak P; Agid Y; Rehncrona S; Volkmann J; Kulisevsky J; Obeso JA; Albanese A; Hariz MI; Quinn NP; Speelman JD; Benabid AL; Fraix V; Mendes A; Welter ML; Houeto JL; Cornu P; Dormont D; Tornqvist AL; Ekberg R; Schnitzler A; Timmermann L; Wojtecki L; Gironell A; Rodriguez-Oroz MC; Guridi J; Bentivoglio AR; Contarino MF; Romito L; Scerrati M; Janssens M; Lang AE
Institution:	Toronto Western Hospital, Movement Disorders Center, University of Toronto and University Health Network, Toronto, Ontario, Canada. elena.moro@uhn.on.ca
Journal:	Mov Disord. 2010 Apr 15;25(5):578-86.
Abstract Link:	http://www.medifocus.com/abstracts.php?gid=NR013&ID=20213817

156.

A phase I study of aromatic L-amino acid decarboxylase gene therapy for Parkinson's disease.

Authors:	Muramatsu S; Fujimoto K; Kato S; Mizukami H; Asari S; Ikeguchi K; Kawakami T; Urabe M; Kume A; Sato T; Watanabe E; Ozawa K; Nakano I
Institution:	Division of Neurology, Department of Medicine, Jichi Medical University, Tochigi, Japan. muramats@jichi.ac.jp
Journal:	Mol Ther. 2010 Sep;18(9):1731-5. Epub 2010 Jul 6.
Abstract Link:	http://www.medifocus.com/abstracts.php?gid=NR013&ID=20606642

157.

High compliance with rotigotine transdermal patch in the treatment of idiopathic Parkinson's disease.

Authors:	Schnitzler A; Leffers KW; Hack HJ
Institution:	Institute of Clinical Neuroscience and Medical Psychology, Heinrich Heine University, Universitatsstr. 1, Dusseldorf, Germany. schnitza@uni-duesseldorf.de
Journal:	Parkinsonism Relat Disord. 2010 Sep;16(8):513-6. Epub 2010 Jul 4.
Abstract Link:	http://www.medifocus.com/abstracts.php?gid=NR013&ID=20605106

Go to http://www.medifocus.com/links/NR013/0112 for direct online access to the above Abstract Links.

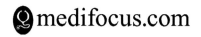

158.

A double-blind, placebo-controlled study to assess the mitochondria-targeted antioxidant MitoQ as a disease-modifying therapy in Parkinson's disease.

Authors:	Snow BJ; Rolfe FL; Lockhart MM; Frampton CM; O'Sullivan JD; Fung V; Smith RA; Murphy MP; Taylor KM
Institution:	Neurology Department, Auckland Hospital, Auckland, New Zealand. bsnow@adhb.govt.nz
Journal:	Mov Disord. 2010 Aug 15;25(11):1670-4.
Abstract Link:	http://www.medifocus.com/abstracts.php?gid=NR013&ID=20568096

159.

The effect of psychotherapy in patients with PD: a controlled study.

Authors:	Sproesser E; Viana MA; Quagliato EM; de Souza EA
Institution:	Department of Neurology, Faculty of Medical Science, University of Campinas - UNICAMP, Caixa postal 6111, CEP-13083 970 Campinas - Sao Paulo, Brazil. erikasproesser@terra.com.br
Journal:	Parkinsonism Relat Disord. 2010 May;16(4):298-300. Epub 2009 Oct 27.
Abstract Link:	http://www.medifocus.com/abstracts.php?gid=NR013&ID=19864172

160.

Initiating levodopa/carbidopa therapy with and without entacapone in early Parkinson disease: the STRIDE-PD study.

Authors:	Stocchi F; Rascol O; Kieburtz K; Poewe W; Jankovic J; Tolosa E; Barone P; Lang AE; Olanow CW
Institution:	Institute of Neurology, IRCCS San Raffaele Pisana, Rome, Italy.
Journal:	Ann Neurol. 2010 Jul;68(1):18-27.
Abstract Link:	http://www.medifocus.com/abstracts.php?gid=NR013&ID=20582993

Go to http://www.medifocus.com/links/NR013/0112 for direct online access to the above Abstract Links.

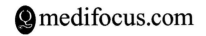

161.

Melevodopa/carbidopa effervescent formulation in the treatment of motor fluctuations in advanced Parkinson's disease.

Authors:	Stocchi F; Zappia M; Dall'Armi V; Kulisevsky J; Lamberti P; Obeso JA
Institution:	Department of Neuroscience, Institute of Neurology, IRCCS San Raffaele Pisana, Roma, Italy. fabrizio.stocchi@fastwebnet.it
Journal:	Mov Disord. 2010 Sep 15;25(12):1881-7.
Abstract Link:	http://www.medifocus.com/abstracts.php?gid=NR013&ID=20669296

162.

A closer look at unilateral versus bilateral deep brain stimulation: results of the National Institutes of Health COMPARE cohort.

Authors:	Taba HA; Wu SS; Foote KD; Hass CJ; Fernandez HH; Malaty IA; Rodriguez RL; Dai Y; Zeilman PR; Jacobson CE; Okun MS
Institution:	Department of Neurology, University of Forlida Movement Disorders Center, College of Medicine, University of Florida, Gainesville, FL 32611, USA.
Journal:	J Neurosurg. 2010 Dec;113(6):1224-9. Epub 2010 Sep 17.
Abstract Link:	http://www.medifocus.com/abstracts.php?gid=NR013&ID=20849215

163.

Pathological gambling in Parkinson disease is reduced by amantadine.

Authors:	Thomas A; Bonanni L; Gambi F; Di Iorio A; Onofrj M
Institution:	Department of Neurology, University G. d'Annunzio, Chieti and Pescara, Italy.
Journal:	Ann Neurol. 2010 Sep;68(3):400-4.
Abstract Link:	http://www.medifocus.com/abstracts.php?gid=NR013&ID=20687121

Go to http://www.medifocus.com/links/NR013/0112 for direct online access to the above Abstract Links.

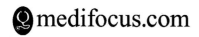

164.

Aspiration and swallowing in Parkinson disease and rehabilitation with EMST: a randomized trial.

Authors:	Troche MS; Okun MS; Rosenbek JC; Musson N; Fernandez HH; Rodriguez R; Romrell J; Pitts T; Wheeler-Hegland KM; Sapienza CM
Institution:	PO Box 117420, University of Florida, Gainesville, FL 32611, USA. michi81@ufl.edu
Journal:	Neurology. 2010 Nov 23;75(21):1912-9.
Abstract Link:	http://www.medifocus.com/abstracts.php?gid=NR013&ID=21098406

165.

Open-labeled study of unilateral autologous bone-marrow-derived mesenchymal stem cell transplantation in Parkinson's disease.

Authors:	Venkataramana NK; Kumar SK; Balaraju S; Radhakrishnan RC; Bansal A; Dixit A; Rao DK; Das M; Jan M; Gupta PK; Totey SM
Institution:	Advanced Neuroscience Institute, BGS-Global Hospital, Bangalore, India. drnkvr@gmail.com
Journal:	Transl Res. 2010 Feb;155(2):62-70. Epub 2009 Aug 6.
Abstract Link:	http://www.medifocus.com/abstracts.php?gid=NR013&ID=20129486

166.

Onset of dyskinesia with adjunct ropinirole prolonged-release or additional levodopa in early Parkinson's disease.

Authors:	Watts RL; Lyons KE; Pahwa R; Sethi K; Stern M; Hauser RA; Olanow W; Gray AM; Adams B; Earl NL
Institution:	Department of Neurology, University of Alabama at Birmingham, Birmingham, Alabama 35294-0017, USA. rlwatts@uab.edu
Journal:	Mov Disord. 2010 May 15;25(7):858-66.
Abstract Link:	http://www.medifocus.com/abstracts.php?gid=NR013&ID=20461803

Go to http://www.medifocus.com/links/NR013/0112 for direct online access to the above Abstract Links.

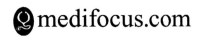

167.

Atomoxetine for depression and other neuropsychiatric symptoms in Parkinson disease.

Authors:	Weintraub D; Mavandadi S; Mamikonyan E; Siderowf AD; Duda JE; Hurtig HI; Colcher A; Horn SS; Nazem S; Ten Have TR; Stern MB
Institution:	Department of Psychiatry, University of Pennsylvania, Philadelphia, USA. daniel.weintraub@uphs.upenn.edu
Journal:	Neurology. 2010 Aug 3;75(5):448-55.
Abstract Link:	http://www.medifocus.com/abstracts.php?gid=NR013&ID=20679638

168.

Deep brain stimulation plus best medical therapy versus best medical therapy alone for advanced Parkinson's disease (PD SURG trial): a randomised, open-label trial.

Authors:	Williams A; Gill S; Varma T; Jenkinson C; Quinn N; Mitchell R; Scott R; Ives N; Rick C; Daniels J; Patel S; Wheatley K
Institution:	Queen Elizabeth Hospital, Birmingham, Birmingham, UK.
Journal:	Lancet Neurol. 2010 Jun;9(6):581-91. Epub 2010 Apr 29.
Abstract Link:	http://www.medifocus.com/abstracts.php?gid=NR013&ID=20434403

169.

Long-term antidyskinetic efficacy of amantadine in Parkinson's disease.

Authors:	Wolf E; Seppi K; Katzenschlager R; Hochschorner G; Ransmayr G; Schwingenschuh P; Ott E; Kloiber I; Haubenberger D; Auff E; Poewe W
Institution:	Department of Neurology, Medical University Innsbruck, Innsbruck, Austria.
Journal:	Mov Disord. 2010 Jul 30;25(10):1357-63.
Abstract Link:	http://www.medifocus.com/abstracts.php?gid=NR013&ID=20198649

Go to http://www.medifocus.com/links/NR013/0112 for direct online access to the above Abstract Links.

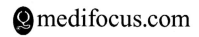
170.

Urate as a predictor of the rate of clinical decline in Parkinson disease.

Authors:	Ascherio A; LeWitt PA; Xu K; Eberly S; Watts A; Matson WR; Marras C; Kieburtz K; Rudolph A; Bogdanov MB; Schwid SR; Tennis M; Tanner CM; Beal MF; Lang AE; Oakes D; Fahn S; Shoulson I; Schwarzschild MA
Institution:	Departments of Nutrition and Epidemiology, Harvard School of Public Health, Boston, Massachusetts, USA.
Journal:	Arch Neurol. 2009 Dec;66(12):1460-8. Epub .
Abstract Link:	http://www.medifocus.com/abstracts.php?gid=NR013&ID=19822770

171.

Safety study of 50 Hz repetitive transcranial magnetic stimulation in patients with Parkinson's disease.

Authors:	Benninger DH; Lomarev M; Wassermann EM; Lopez G; Houdayer E; Fasano RE; Dang N; Hallett M
Institution:	Human Motor Control Section, Medical Neurology Branch, National Institute of Neurological Disorders and Stroke, National Institutes of Health, Building 10 Room 7D42 (MSC1428), Center Drive, Bethesda, MD 20892, USA. benningerd@ninds.nih.gov
Journal:	Clin Neurophysiol. 2009 Apr;120(4):809-15. Epub 2009 Mar 14.
Abstract Link:	http://www.medifocus.com/abstracts.php?gid=NR013&ID=19285918

172.

Novel challenges to gait in Parkinson's disease: the effect of concurrent music in single- and dual-task contexts.

Authors:	Brown LA; de Bruin N; Doan JB; Suchowersky O; Hu B
Institution:	Department of Kinesiology, University of Lethbridge, Lethbridge, Alberta, Canada. l.brown@uleth.ca
Journal:	Arch Phys Med Rehabil. 2009 Sep;90(9):1578-83.
Abstract Link:	http://www.medifocus.com/abstracts.php?gid=NR013&ID=19735787

Go to http://www.medifocus.com/links/NR013/0112 for direct online access to the above Abstract Links.

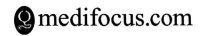

173.

Safety and tolerability of putaminal AADC gene therapy for Parkinson disease.

Authors: Christine CW; Starr PA; Larson PS; Eberling JL; Jagust WJ; Hawkins RA; VanBrocklin HF; Wright JF; Bankiewicz KS; Aminoff MJ

Institution: Department of Neurology, University of California, San Francisco, CA 94143-0114, USA.

Journal: Neurology. 2009 Nov 17;73(20):1662-9. Epub 2009 Oct 14.

Abstract Link: http://www.medifocus.com/abstracts.php?gid=NR013&ID=19828868

174.

Long-term superiority of subthalamic nucleus stimulation over pallidotomy in Parkinson disease.

Authors: Esselink RA; de Bie RM; de Haan RJ; Lenders MW; Nijssen PC; van Laar T; Schuurman PR; Bosch DA; Speelman JD

Institution: Departments of Neurology and Geriatrics, Radboud University Nijmegen Medical Centre, Donders Institute for Brain, Cognition, and Behaviour, PO Box 9101, 6500 HB Nijmegen, the Netherlands. r.esselink@neuro.umcn.nl

Journal: Neurology. 2009 Jul 14;73(2):151-3.

Abstract Link: **ABSTRACT NOT AVAILABLE**

175.

Subthalamic nucleus stimulation in Parkinson disease induces apathy: a PET study.

Authors: Le Jeune F; Drapier D; Bourguignon A; Peron J; Mesbah H; Drapier S; Sauleau P; Haegelen C; Travers D; Garin E; Malbert CH; Millet B; Verin M

Institution: Service de Medecine Nucleaire, Centre Eugene Marquis, Renne, France.

Journal: Neurology. 2009 Nov 24;73(21):1746-51.

Abstract Link: http://www.medifocus.com/abstracts.php?gid=NR013&ID=19933975

Go to http://www.medifocus.com/links/NR013/0112 for direct online access to the above Abstract Links.

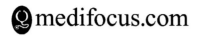

176.

A double-blind, delayed-start trial of rasagiline in Parkinson's disease.

Authors:	Olanow CW; Rascol O; Hauser R; Feigin PD; Jankovic J; Lang A; Langston W; Melamed E; Poewe W; Stocchi F; Tolosa E
Institution:	Department of Neurology and Neuroscience, Mount Sinai School of Medicine, New York, NY 10029, USA. warren.olanow@mssm.edu
Journal:	N Engl J Med. 2009 Sep 24;361(13):1268-78.
Abstract Link:	http://www.medifocus.com/abstracts.php?gid=NR013&ID=19776408

177.

Determinants of the timing of symptomatic treatment in early Parkinson disease: The National Institutes of Health Exploratory Trials in Parkinson Disease (NET-PD) Experience.

Authors:	Parashos SA; Swearingen CJ; Biglan KM; Bodis-Wollner I; Liang GS; Ross GW; Tilley BC; Shulman LM
Institution:	Struthers Parkinson's Center, 6701 Country Club Dr, Golden Valley, MN 55427, USA. sotirios.parashos@mpls-clinic.com
Journal:	Arch Neurol. 2009 Sep;66(9):1099-104. Epub 2009 Jul 13.
Abstract Link:	http://www.medifocus.com/abstracts.php?gid=NR013&ID=19597081

178.

Occupation and risk of parkinsonism: a multicenter case-control study.

Authors:	Tanner CM; Ross GW; Jewell SA; Hauser RA; Jankovic J; Factor SA; Bressman S; Deligtisch A; Marras C; Lyons KE; Bhudhikanok GS; Roucoux DF; Meng C; Abbott RD; Langston JW
Institution:	Department of Clinical Research, The Parkinson's Institute, Sunnyvale, California 94085, USA. CTanner@thepi.org
Journal:	Arch Neurol. 2009 Sep;66(9):1106-13.
Abstract Link:	http://www.medifocus.com/abstracts.php?gid=NR013&ID=19752299

Go to http://www.medifocus.com/links/NR013/0112 for direct online access to the above Abstract Links.

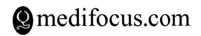

179.

Stridor and dysphagia associated with subthalamic nucleus stimulation in Parkinson disease.

Authors:	Fagbami OY; Donato AA
Institution:	Department of Internal Medicine, The Reading Hospital and Medical Center, West Reading, Pennsylvania 19612, USA. fagbamio@readinghospital.org
Journal:	J Neurosurg. 2011 Nov;115(5):1005-6. Epub 2011 Aug 5.
Abstract Link:	http://www.medifocus.com/abstracts.php?gid=NR013&ID=21819188

180.

The relevance of age and disease duration for intervention with subthalamic nucleus deep brain stimulation surgery in Parkinson disease.

Authors:	Parent B; Awan N; Berman SB; Suski V; Moore R; Crammond D; Kondziolka D
Institution:	Department of Neurological Surgery, and Center for Brain Function and Behavior, University of Pittsburgh Medical Center, Pittsburgh, Pennsylvania 15213, USA.
Journal:	J Neurosurg. 2011 Apr;114(4):927-31. Epub 2010 Nov 26.
Abstract Link:	http://www.medifocus.com/abstracts.php?gid=NR013&ID=21110713

181.

Effects of subthalamic stimulation on speech of consecutive patients with Parkinson disease.

Authors:	Tripoliti E; Zrinzo L; Martinez-Torres I; Frost E; Pinto S; Foltynie T; Holl E; Petersen E; Roughton M; Hariz MI; Limousin P
Institution:	Sobell Department, Unit of Functional Neurosurgery, UCL Institute of Neurology, Box 146, Queen Square, London, WC1N 3BG, UK. e.tripoliti@ion.ucl.ac.uk
Journal:	Neurology. 2011 Jan 4;76(1):80-6. Epub 2010 Nov 10.
Abstract Link:	http://www.medifocus.com/abstracts.php?gid=NR013&ID=21068426

Go to http://www.medifocus.com/links/NR013/0112 for direct online access to the above Abstract Links.

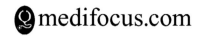

182.

Subthalamic nucleus stimulation for Parkinson disease with severe medication-induced hallucinations or delusions.

Authors: Umemura A; Oka Y; Okita K; Matsukawa N; Yamada K

Institution: Department of Neurosurgery, Nagoya City University Graduate School of Medicine, 1 Kawasumi, Mizuho-ku, Nagoya 467-8601, Japan. aume@med.nagoya-cu.ac.jp

Journal: J Neurosurg. 2011 Jun;114(6):1701-5. Epub 2011 Mar 4.

Abstract Link: http://www.medifocus.com/abstracts.php?gid=NR013&ID=21375379

183.

Cognitive and neuropsychiatric effects of subthalamotomy for Parkinson's disease.

Authors: Bickel S; Alvarez L; Macias R; Pavon N; Leon M; Fernandez C; Houghton DJ; Salazar S; Rodriguez-Oroz MC; Juncos J; Guridi J; Delong M; Obeso JA; Litvan I

Institution: Division of Movement Disorders, Department of Neurology, University of Louisville School of Medicine, Frazier Rehab Neuroscience Institute, 220 Abraham Flexner Way, Ste 1503, Louisville, KY 40202, USA.

Journal: Parkinsonism Relat Disord. 2010 Sep;16(8):535-9. Epub 2010 Jul 21.

Abstract Link: http://www.medifocus.com/abstracts.php?gid=NR013&ID=20650671

184.

Early versus delayed bilateral subthalamic deep brain stimulation for parkinson's disease: a decision analysis.

Authors: Espay AJ; Vaughan JE; Marras C; Fowler R; Eckman MH

Institution: Department of Neurology, Movement Disorders Center, The Neuroscience Institute, University of Cincinnati, Cincinnati, Ohio 45267-0525, USA. alberto.espay@uc.edu

Journal: Mov Disord. 2010 Jul 30;25(10):1456-63.

Abstract Link: http://www.medifocus.com/abstracts.php?gid=NR013&ID=20629150

Go to http://www.medifocus.com/links/NR013/0112 for direct online access to the above Abstract Links.

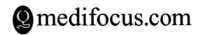

185.

Motor and cognitive outcome in patients with Parkinson's disease 8 years after subthalamic implants.

Authors:	Fasano A; Romito LM; Daniele A; Piano C; Zinno M; Bentivoglio AR; Albanese A
Institution:	Istituto di Neurologia, Universita Cattolica del Sacro Cuore, Rome, Italy.
Journal:	Brain. 2010 Sep;133(9):2664-76.
Abstract Link:	http://www.medifocus.com/abstracts.php?gid=NR013&ID=20802207

186.

Pallidal stimulation in advanced Parkinson's patients with contraindications for subthalamic stimulation.

Authors:	Rouaud T; Dondaine T; Drapier S; Haegelen C; Lallement F; Peron J; Raoul S; Sauleau P; Verin M
Institution:	Department of Neurology, University Hospital of Rennes, Rennes, France.
Journal:	Mov Disord. 2010 Sep 15;25(12):1839-46.
Abstract Link:	http://www.medifocus.com/abstracts.php?gid=NR013&ID=20568094

187.

A meta-regression of the long-term effects of deep brain stimulation on balance and gait in PD.

Authors:	St George RJ; Nutt JG; Burchiel KJ; Horak FB
Institution:	Department of Neurology, Oregon Health & Sciences University, 505 NW 185 Avenue, Beaverton, OR 97006, USA. stgeorgr@ohsu.edu
Journal:	Neurology. 2010 Oct 5;75(14):1292-9.
Abstract Link:	http://www.medifocus.com/abstracts.php?gid=NR013&ID=20921515

Go to http://www.medifocus.com/links/NR013/0112 for direct online access to the above Abstract Links.

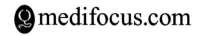

188.

Subthalamic nucleus stimulation influences expression and suppression of impulsive behaviour in Parkinson's disease.

Authors:	Wylie SA; Ridderinkhof KR; Elias WJ; Frysinger RC; Bashore TR; Downs KE; van Wouwe NC; van den Wildenberg WP
Institution:	Neurology Department, University of Virginia Health Systems, Charlottesville, VA 22908, USA. saw6n@virginia.edu
Journal:	Brain. 2010 Dec;133(Pt 12):3611-24. Epub 2010 Sep 22.
Abstract Link:	http://www.medifocus.com/abstracts.php?gid=NR013&ID=20861152

189.

Subthalamic nucleus stimulation does not cause deterioration of preexisting hallucinations in Parkinson's disease patients.

Authors:	Yoshida F; Miyagi Y; Kishimoto J; Morioka T; Murakami N; Hashiguchi K; Samura K; Sakae N; Yamasaki R; Kawaguchi M; Sasaki T
Institution:	Department of Neurosurgery, Kyushu University, Higashi-ku, Fukuoka, Japan.
Journal:	Stereotact Funct Neurosurg. 2009;87(1):45-9. Epub 2009 Jan 28.
Abstract Link:	http://www.medifocus.com/abstracts.php?gid=NR013&ID=19174620

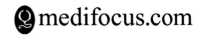

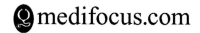

NOTES

Use this page for taking notes as you review your Guidebook

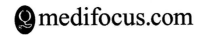

4 - Centers of Research

This section of your *MediFocus Guidebook* is a unique directory of doctors, researchers, medical centers, and research institutions with specialized research interest, and in many cases, clinical expertise in the management of this specific medical condition. The *Centers of Research* directory is a valuable resource for quickly identifying and locating leading medical authorities and medical institutions within the United States and other countries that are considered to be at the forefront in clinical research and treatment of this disorder.

Use the *Centers of Research* directory to contact, consult, or network with leading experts in the field and to locate a hospital or medical center that can help you.

The following information is provided in the *Centers of Research* directory:

- **Geographic Location**

  - United States: the information is divided by individual states listed in alphabetical order. Not all states may be included.

  - Other Countries: information is presented for select countries worldwide listed in alphabetical order. Not all countries may be included.

- **Names of Authors**

  - Select names of individual authors (doctors, researchers, or other health-care professionals) with specialized research interest, and in many cases, clinical expertise in the management of this specific medical condition, who have recently published articles in leading medical journals about the condition.

  - E-mail addresses for individual authors, if listed on their specific publications, is also provided.

- **Institutional Affiliations**

  - Next to each individual author's name is their **institutional affiliation** (hospital, medical center, or research institution) where the study was conducted as listed in their publication(s).

- In many cases, information about the specific **department** within the medical institution where the individual author was located at the time the study was conducted is also provided.

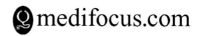

Centers of Research

United States

AL - Alabama

Name of Author	Institutional Affiliation
Bickel CS	Department of Physical Therapy, University of Alabama, Birmingham, Birmingham, AL, USA. mford@uab.edu
Earl NL	Department of Neurology, University of Alabama at Birmingham, Birmingham, Alabama 35294-0017, USA. rlwatts@uab.edu
Ford MP	Department of Physical Therapy, University of Alabama, Birmingham, Birmingham, AL, USA. mford@uab.edu
Watts RL	Department of Neurology, University of Alabama at Birmingham, Birmingham, Alabama 35294-0017, USA. rlwatts@uab.edu

CA - California

Name of Author	Institutional Affiliation
Aminoff MJ	Department of Neurology, University of California, San Francisco, CA 94143-0114, USA.
Bronstein J	Movement Disorders Program, UCLA Department of Neurology, 300 UCLA Medical Plaza Ste. B200, Los Angeles, CA 90095, USA. efarag@mednet.ucla.edu
Bronstein JM	University of California, Los Angeles, School of Medicine, Department of Neurology, 710 Westwood Plaza, Los Angeles, CA 90095, USA. jbronste@ucla.edu
Christine CW	Department of Neurology, University of California, San Francisco, CA 94143-0114, USA.
DeLong MR	University of California, Los Angeles, School of Medicine, Department of Neurology, 710 Westwood Plaza, Los Angeles, CA 90095, USA. jbronste@ucla.edu

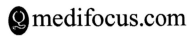

Farag ES	Movement Disorders Program, UCLA Department of Neurology, 300 UCLA Medical Plaza Ste. B200, Los Angeles, CA 90095, USA. efarag@mednet.ucla.edu
Hitzeman N	Sutter Health Family Medicine Residency Program, Sacramento, CA, USA. hitzemn@sutterhealth.org
Langston JW	Department of Clinical Research, The Parkinson's Institute, Sunnyvale, California 94085, USA. CTanner@thepi.org
Lo RY	The Parkinson's Institute and Clinical Center, Sunnyvale, CA 94085, USA.
Marks WJ Jr	Department of Neurology, University of California San Francisco, San Francisco, CA, USA.
Olanow CW	Department of Neurology, University of California San Francisco, San Francisco, CA, USA.
Rafii F	Sutter Health Family Medicine Residency Program, Sacramento, CA, USA. hitzemn@sutterhealth.org
Tanner CM	Department of Clinical Research, The Parkinson's Institute, Sunnyvale, California 94085, USA. CTanner@thepi.org
Van Den Eeden SK	The Parkinson's Institute and Clinical Center, Sunnyvale, CA 94085, USA.

CO - Colorado

Name of Author	Institutional Affiliation
Bainbridge JL	Department of Clinical Pharmacy, University of Colorado Denver, Aurora, Colorado 80045, USA. jacci.bainbridge@uchsc.edu
Ruscin JM	Department of Clinical Pharmacy, University of Colorado Denver, Aurora, Colorado 80045, USA. jacci.bainbridge@uchsc.edu
Schenkman M	Department of Physical Medicine and Rehabilitation, School of Medicine, University of Colorado, Aurora, CO 80045, USA. margaret.schenkman@ucdenver.edu
Wagenaar R	Department of Physical Medicine and Rehabilitation, School of Medicine, University of Colorado, Aurora, CO 80045, USA. margaret.schenkman@ucdenver.edu

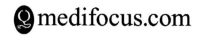
medifocus.com

FL - Florida

Name of Author	Institutional Affiliation
Fernandez HH	College of Medicine, University of Florida, Gainesville, FL 32610, USA.
Katzen H	Division of Neuropsychology, Department of Neurology, University of Miami, Miller School of Medicine, Miami, FL 33136, USA. hkatzen@med.miami.edu
LaPointe LL	Florida State University, Tallahassee, FL, USA. lllapointe@fsu.edu
Leibner J	College of Medicine, University of Florida, Gainesville, FL 32610, USA.
Levin B	Division of Neuropsychology, Department of Neurology, University of Miami, Miller School of Medicine, Miami, FL 33136, USA. hkatzen@med.miami.edu
Maitland CG	Florida State University, Tallahassee, FL, USA. lllapointe@fsu.edu
Okun MS	Department of Neurology, University of Forlida Movement Disorders Center, College of Medicine, University of Florida, Gainesville, FL 32611, USA.
Sapienza CM	PO Box 117420, University of Florida, Gainesville, FL 32611, USA. michi81@ufl.edu
Taba HA	Department of Neurology, University of Forlida Movement Disorders Center, College of Medicine, University of Florida, Gainesville, FL 32611, USA.
Troche MS	PO Box 117420, University of Florida, Gainesville, FL 32611, USA. michi81@ufl.edu
Weiner WJ	University of South Florida, Tampa, USA.
Zesiewicz TA	University of South Florida, Tampa, USA.

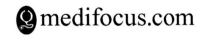

GA - Georgia

Name of Author	Institutional Affiliation
Evatt ML	Department of Neurology, Emory University School of Medicine, 1841 Clifton Rd NE, Atlanta, GA 30329, USA. mevatt@emory.edu
Tangpricha V	Department of Neurology, Emory University School of Medicine, 1841 Clifton Rd NE, Atlanta, GA 30329, USA. mevatt@emory.edu

IA - Iowa

Name of Author	Institutional Affiliation
Dawson JD	Department of Neurology, University of Iowa, Carver College of Medicine, Iowa City, IA 52242, USA. ergun-uc@uiowa.edu
Follett KA	Iowa City Veterans Affairs Medical Center, Iowa City, USA.
Growdon JC	Department of Neurology, University of Iowa, Carver College of Medicine, 200 Hawkins Drive-2RCP, Iowa City, IA 52242, USA. ergun-uc@uiowa.edu
Reda DJ	Iowa City Veterans Affairs Medical Center, Iowa City, USA.
Uc EY	Department of Neurology, University of Iowa, Carver College of Medicine, Iowa City, IA 52242, USA. ergun-uc@uiowa.edu

IL - Illinois

Name of Author	Institutional Affiliation
Aegesen AL	Northwestern University, Rehabilitation Institute of Chicago, Illinois, USA.
Eller T	NorthShore University HealthSystem, Evanston Hospital, Evanston, Illinois, USA.

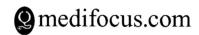

Goetz CG	Movement Disorders Section, Department of Neurological Sciences, Rush University Medical Center, Suite 1106, Chicago, IL 60612, USA. cgoetz@rush.edu
Marciniak CM	Northwestern University, Rehabilitation Institute of Chicago, Illinois, USA.
Simuni T	Department of Neurology, Northwestern University, Parkinson's Disease and Movement Disorders Center, Chicago, Ill, USA. tsimuni@nmff.org
Stebbins GT	Movement Disorders Section, Department of Neurological Sciences, Rush University Medical Center, Suite 1106, Chicago, IL 60612, USA. cgoetz@rush.edu
Weintraub D	Department of Neurology, Northwestern University, Parkinson's Disease and Movement Disorders Center, Chicago, Ill, USA. tsimuni@nmff.org

IN - Indiana

Name of Author	Institutional Affiliation
Combs SA	Krannert School of Physical Therapy, University of Indianapolis, 1400 E Hanna Ave, Indianapolis, IN 46227, USA. scombs@uindy.edu
Davis LL	School of Nursing, Indiana University, Indianapolis, IN, USA. smclenno@iupui.edu
McLennon SM	School of Nursing, Indiana University, Indianapolis, IN, USA. smclenno@iupui.edu
Schaneman K	Krannert School of Physical Therapy, University of Indianapolis, 1400 E Hanna Ave, Indianapolis, IN 46227, USA. scombs@uindy.edu

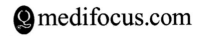
KS - Kansas

Name of Author	Institutional Affiliation
Eng ML	Department of Pharmacy Practice, University of Kansas School of Pharmacy, Kansas City, Kansas 66160, USA. meng@kumc.edu
Welty TE	Department of Pharmacy Practice, University of Kansas School of Pharmacy, Kansas City, Kansas 66160, USA. meng@kumc.edu

KY - Kentucky

Name of Author	Institutional Affiliation
Bickel S	Division of Movement Disorders, Department of Neurology, University of Louisville School of Medicine, Frazier Rehab Neuroscience Institute, 220 Abraham Flexner Way, Ste 1503, Louisville, KY 40202, USA.
Litvan I	Division of Movement Disorders, Department of Neurology, University of Louisville School of Medicine, Frazier Rehab Neuroscience Institute, 220 Abraham Flexner Way, Ste 1503, Louisville, KY 40202, USA.

LA - Louisiana

Name of Author	Institutional Affiliation
Jankovic J	Diana Helis Henry Medical Research Foundation, New Orleans, LA, USA.
Pan T	Diana Helis Henry Medical Research Foundation, New Orleans, LA, USA.
Rajasankar S	School of Medicine, LSUHSC, New Orleans, LA 70112, USA. sankar_surendran@yahoo.com
Surendran S	School of Medicine, LSUHSC, New Orleans, LA 70112, USA. sankar_surendran@yahoo.com

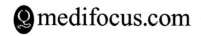 medifocus.com

MA - Massachussetts

Name of Author	Institutional Affiliation
Ascherio A	Department of Epidemiology, Harvard School of Public Health, Boston, Massachusetts, USA. hgardener@med.miami.edu
Bajaj A	Channing Laboratory, Department of Medicine, Brigham and Women's Hospital and Harvard Medical School, 181 Longwood Avenue, Boston, MA 02115, USA. n2baj@channing.harvard.edu
Bortan E	Department of Neurology, Tufts University School of Medicine, Lahey Clinic, Burlington, MA 01805, USA. leegwa00@lahey.org
Gagne JJ	Department of Epidemiology, Harvard School of Public Health, Boston, MA, USA. jgagne1@partners.org
Gao X	Channing Laboratory, Department of Medicine, Brigham and Women's Hospital, and Harvard Medical School, 181 Longwood Ave., Boston, MA 02115, USA. xiang.gao@channing.harvard.edu
Gardener H	Department of Epidemiology, Harvard School of Public Health, Boston, Massachusetts, USA. hgardener@med.miami.edu
Hersh BP	Department of Neurology, Harvard Vanguard Medical Associates, Boston, Massachusetts 02215, USA. bonnie_hersh@vmed.org
Leegwater-Kim J	Department of Neurology, Tufts University School of Medicine, Lahey Clinic, Burlington, MA 01805, USA. leegwa00@lahey.org
Power MC	Department of Epidemiology, Harvard School of Public Health, Boston, MA, USA. jgagne1@partners.org
Schernhammer ES	Channing Laboratory, Department of Medicine, Brigham and Women's Hospital and Harvard Medical School, 181 Longwood Avenue, Boston, MA 02115, USA. n2baj@channing.harvard.edu
Schwarzschild MA	Departments of Nutrition and Epidemiology, Harvard School of Public Health, Boston, Massachusetts, USA.

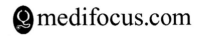

Stacy M — Department of Neurology, Harvard Vanguard Medical Associates, Boston, Massachusetts 02215, USA. bonnie_hersh@vmed.org

MD - Maryland

Name of Author	Institutional Affiliation
Benninger DH	Medical Neurology Branch, National Institute of Neurological Disorders and Stroke, National Institutes of Health, Bethesda, Maryland 20892, USA. benningerd@ninds.nih.gov
Guilarte TR	Neurotoxicology and Molecular Imaging Laboratory, Department of Environmental Health Sciences, Johns Hopkins Bloomberg School of Public Health, Baltimore, Maryland, USA. trguilarte@columbia.edu
Hallett M	Medical Neurology Branch, National Institute of Neurological Disorders and Stroke, National Institutes of Health, Bethesda, Maryland 20892, USA. benningerd@ninds.nih.gov

MI - Michigan

Name of Author	Institutional Affiliation
Bohnen NI	Department of Radiology, Division of Nuclear Medicine, University of Michigan, Ann Arbor, MI 48109, USA. nbohnen@umich.edu
Frey KA	Department of Radiology, Division of Nuclear Medicine, University of Michigan, Ann Arbor, MI 48109, USA. nbohnen@umich.edu

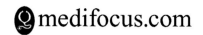

MN - Minnesota

Name of Author	Institutional Affiliation
Ahlskog JE	Department of Health Sciences Research, Mayo Clinic, Rochester, MN 55905, USA.
Parashos SA	Struthers Parkinson's Center, 6701 Country Club Dr, Golden Valley, MN 55427, USA. sotirios.parashos@mpls-clinic.com
Rocca WA	Department of Neurology, Mayo Clinic, Rochester, MN 55905, USA.
Savica R	Department of Neurology, Mayo Clinic, Rochester, MN 55905, USA.
Shulman LM	Struthers Parkinson's Center, 6701 Country Club Dr, Golden Valley, MN 55427, USA. sotirios.parashos@mpls-clinic.com

NC - North Carolina

Name of Author	Institutional Affiliation
Blair A	Epidemiology Branch, National Institute of Environmental Health Sciences, 111 T.W. Alexander Dr., PO Box 12233, Mail drop A3-05, Research Triangle Park, NC 27709, USA. chenh2@niehs.nih.gov
Chen H	Epidemiology Branch, National Institute of Environmental Health Sciences, 111 T.W. Alexander Drive, Research Triangle Park, NC 27709, USA.
Liu R	Epidemiology Branch, National Institute of Environmental Health Sciences, Research Triangle Park, NC 27709, USA.
Xu Q	Epidemiology Branch, National Institute of Environmental Health Sciences, 111 T.W. Alexander Drive, Research Triangle Park, NC 27709, USA.

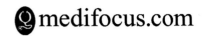

NJ - New Jersey

Name of Author	Institutional Affiliation
Dobkin RD	Department of Psychiatry, University of Medicine and Dentistry of New Jersey-Robert Wood Johnson Medical School, Piscataway, USA. dobkinro@umdnj.edu
Friedman J	Department of Psychiatry, University of Medicine and Dentistry of New Jersey-Robert Wood Johnson Medical School, Piscataway, USA. dobkinro@umdnj.edu
German DC	Robert Wood Johnson Medical School, Piscataway, New Jersey, USA. jricha3@eohsi.rutgers.edu
Hyer L	Department of Psychiatry, Robert Wood Johnson Medical School, Piscataway, New Jersey 08854, USA. menza@umdnj.edu
Menza M	Department of Psychiatry, Robert Wood Johnson Medical School, Piscataway, New Jersey 08854, USA. menza@umdnj.edu
Richardson JR	Robert Wood Johnson Medical School, Piscataway, New Jersey, USA. jricha3@eohsi.rutgers.edu
Troster A	Department of Psychiatry, UMDNJ, Robert Wood Johnson Medical School, D317, 675 Hoes Lane, Piscataway, NJ 08854, USA. dobkinro@umdnj.edu

NY - New York

Name of Author	Institutional Affiliation
Bodis-Wollner IG	Department of Neurology, State University of New York Downstate Medical Center, Brooklyn, NY 11203, USA.
Eidelberg D	Center for Neurosciences, The Feinstein Institute for Medical Research, Manhasset, New York 11030, USA. yma@nshs.edu
Hajee ME	Department of Neurology, State University of New York Downstate Medical Center, Brooklyn, NY 11203, USA.
Kieburtz K	Department of Neurology and Neuroscience, Mount Sinai School of Medicine, New York, New York 10029, USA. warren.olanow@mssm.edu

162 *© Copyright 2012 MediFocus Guide from Medifocus.com, Inc.www.medifocus.com* *(800) 965-3002*

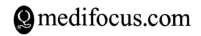

Kiernan HA	Department of Orthopaedic Surgery, Center for Hip and Knee Replacement, New York-Presbyterian Hospital at Columbia University Medical Center, New York, NY, USA.
Ma Y	Center for Neurosciences, The Feinstein Institute for Medical Research, Manhasset, New York 11030, USA. yma@nshs.edu
Macaulay W	Department of Orthopaedic Surgery, Center for Hip and Knee Replacement, New York-Presbyterian Hospital at Columbia University Medical Center, New York, NY, USA.
Olanow CW	Department of Neurology and Neuroscience, Mount Sinai School of Medicine, New York, NY 10029, USA. warren.olanow@mssm.edu
Tolosa E	Department of Neurology and Neuroscience, Mount Sinai School of Medicine, New York, NY 10029, USA. warren.olanow@mssm.edu

OH - Ohio

Name of Author	Institutional Affiliation
Eckman MH	Department of Neurology, Movement Disorders Center, The Neuroscience Institute, University of Cincinnati, Cincinnati, Ohio 45267-0525, USA. alberto.espay@uc.edu
Espay AJ	Department of Neurology, University of Cincinnati, Cincinnati, OH 45267-0525, USA. alberto.espay@uc.edu
Shukla R	Department of Neurology, University of Cincinnati, Cincinnati, OH 45267-0525, USA. alberto.espay@uc.edu

OR - Oregon

Name of Author	Institutional Affiliation
Chung KA	Department of Neurology, Oregon Health & Science University, Portland, OR, USA. chungka@ohsu.edu
Horak FB	Department of Neurology, Oregon Health & Sciences University, 505 NW 185 Avenue, Beaverton, OR 97006, USA. stgeorgr@ohsu.edu

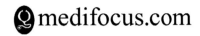

Lou JS	Oregon Health & Science University, Portland, Oregon, USA. Louja@ohsu.edu
St George RJ	Department of Neurology, Oregon Health & Sciences University, 505 NW 185 Avenue, Beaverton, OR 97006, USA. stgeorgr@ohsu.edu

PA - Pennsylvania

Name of Author	Institutional Affiliation
Donato AA	Department of Internal Medicine, The Reading Hospital and Medical Center, West Reading, Pennsylvania 19612, USA. fagbamio@readinghospital.org
Fagbami OY	Department of Internal Medicine, The Reading Hospital and Medical Center, West Reading, Pennsylvania 19612, USA. fagbamio@readinghospital.org
Galpern WR	Department of Pathology, Anatomy and Cell Biology, Thomas Jefferson University, 1020 Locust Street, 521 JAH, Philadelphia, PA 19107, USA. jay.schneider@jefferson.edu
Hurtig HI	Parkinson's Disease and Movement Disorders Center, Department of Neurology, University of Pennsylvania, Philadelphia, PA 19107, USA.
Kales HC	Department of Psychiatry, University of Pennsylvania, Philadelphia, PA 19104, USA. daniel.weintraub@uphs.upenn.edu
Kondziolka D	Department of Neurological Surgery, and Center for Brain Function and Behavior, University of Pittsburgh Medical Center, Pittsburgh, Pennsylvania 15213, USA.
Morley JF	Parkinson's Disease and Movement Disorders Center, Department of Neurology, University of Pennsylvania, Philadelphia, PA 19107, USA.
Parent B	Department of Neurological Surgery, and Center for Brain Function and Behavior, University of Pittsburgh Medical Center, Pittsburgh, Pennsylvania 15213, USA.
Schneider JS	Department of Pathology, Anatomy and Cell Biology, Thomas Jefferson University, 1020 Locust Street, 521 JAH, Philadelphia, PA 19107, USA. jay.schneider@jefferson.edu

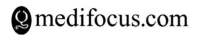

| Stern MB | Department of Psychiatry, University of Pennsylvania, Philadelphia, USA. daniel.weintraub@uphs.upenn.edu |
| Weintraub D | Department of Psychiatry, University of Pennsylvania, Philadelphia, USA. daniel.weintraub@uphs.upenn.edu |

RI - Rhode Island

Name of Author	**Institutional Affiliation**
Friedman JH	Alpert Medical School, Brown University, Providence, RI 02886, USA.
Thomas AA	Alpert Medical School, Brown University, Providence, RI 02886, USA.

TN - Tennessee

| **Name of Author** | **Institutional Affiliation** |
| Pfeiffer RF | Department of Neurology, University of Tennessee Health Science Center, 855 Monroe Avenue, Memphis, TN 38163, USA. rpfeiffer@uthsc.edu |

VA - Virginia

Name of Author	**Institutional Affiliation**
Wylie SA	Neurology Department, University of Virginia Health Systems, Charlottesville, VA 22908, USA. saw6n@virginia.edu
van den Wildenberg WP	Neurology Department, University of Virginia Health Systems, Charlottesville, VA 22908, USA. saw6n@virginia.edu

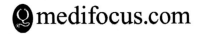

WA - Washington

Name of Author	Institutional Affiliation
Dobbins EK	Elder Services, Spokane, Washington, USA. lindy_wood@wsu.edu
Wood LD	Elder Services, Spokane, Washington, USA. lindy_wood@wsu.edu

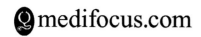
Centers of Research

Other Countries

Australia

Name of Author	Institutional Affiliation
Dissanayaka NN	Neurology Research Centre, Royal Brisbane and Women's Hospital, Brisbane, Australia. n.dissanayaka@griffith.edu.au
Halliday GM	Prince of Wales Medical Research Institute and University of New South Wales, Sydney, Australia. g.halliday@powmri.edu.au
Kerr GK	School of Human Movement Studies, Institute of Health and Biomedical Innovation, Royal Brisbane and Women's Hospital, Queensland, Australia. g.kerr@qut.edu.au
McCann H	Prince of Wales Medical Research Institute and University of New South Wales, Sydney, Australia. g.halliday@powmri.edu.au
McGinley JL	Melbourne School of Health Sciences, The University of Melbourne, 200 Berkeley Street, Victoria 3010, Australia. ssoh@unimelb.edu.au
Mellick GD	Neurology Research Centre, Royal Brisbane and Women's Hospital, Brisbane, Australia. n.dissanayaka@griffith.edu.au
Morris ME	School of Health Sciences, University of Melbourne, Melbourne, Australia. dawn.tan.m.l@sgh.com.sg
Murdoch BE	The University of Queensland, Brisbane, Australia. b.murdoch@uq.edu.au
Silburn PA	School of Human Movement Studies, Institute of Health and Biomedical Innovation, Royal Brisbane and Women's Hospital, Queensland, Australia. g.kerr@qut.edu.au
Soh SE	Melbourne School of Health Sciences, The University of Melbourne, 200 Berkeley Street, Victoria 3010, Australia. ssoh@unimelb.edu.au

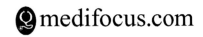

| Tan DM | School of Health Sciences, University of Melbourne, Melbourne, Australia. dawn.tan.m.l@sgh.com.sg |

Austria

Name of Author	Institutional Affiliation
Enzinger C	Paediatric Orthopaedic Unit, Department of Paediatric Surgery, Medical University of Graz, Auenbruggerplatz 34, Graz, A-8036, Austria. martin.spejlik@seznam.cz
Poewe W	Department of Neurology, Medical University Innsbruck, Innsbruck, Austria.
Schapira AH	Innsbruck Medical University, Innsbruck, Austria. werner.poewe@i-med.ac.at
Svehlik M	Paediatric Orthopaedic Unit, Department of Paediatric Surgery, Medical University of Graz, Auenbruggerplatz 34, Graz, A-8036, Austria. martin.spejlik@seznam.cz
Wolf E	Department of Neurology, Medical University Innsbruck, Innsbruck, Austria.

Brazil

Name of Author	Institutional Affiliation
De Araujo DP	Department of Physiology and Pharmacology, Faculty of Medicine, Federal University of Ceara, Brazil.
Sproesser E	Department of Neurology, Faculty of Medical Science, University of Campinas - UNICAMP, Caixa postal 6111, CEP-13083 970 Campinas - Sao Paulo, Brazil. erikasproesser@terra.com.br
Vasconcelos SM	Department of Physiology and Pharmacology, Faculty of Medicine, Federal University of Ceara, Brazil.
de Souza EA	Department of Neurology, Faculty of Medical Science, University of Campinas - UNICAMP, Caixa postal 6111, CEP-13083 970 Campinas - Sao Paulo, Brazil. erikasproesser@terra.com.br

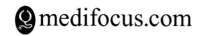

Canada

Name of Author	Institutional Affiliation
Brown LA	Department of Kinesiology, University of Lethbridge, Lethbridge, Alberta, Canada. l.brown@uleth.ca
Hu B	Department of Kinesiology, University of Lethbridge, Lethbridge, Alberta, Canada. l.brown@uleth.ca
Hung SW	Movement Disorders Centre, Toronto Western Hospital and Division of Neurology, University of Toronto, Toronto, Canada.
Jog MS	cMovement Disorders Clinic, London Health Sciences Centre, 339 Windemere Blvd, A 10-026, London, Ontario Canada. asouth4@uwo.ca
Lang AE	Toronto Western Hospital, Movement Disorders Center, University of Toronto and University Health Network, Toronto, Ontario, Canada. elena.moro@uhn.on.ca
Lozano AM	Movement Disorders Centre, Division of Neurology, Department of Medicine, University of Toronto, Toronto Western Hospital, University Health Network,Toronto, ON M5T2S8, Canada. elena.moro@uhn.on.ca
Moro E	Toronto Western Hospital, Movement Disorders Center, University of Toronto and University Health Network, Toronto, Ontario, Canada. elena.moro@uhn.on.ca
Rajput A	Division of Neurology, Department of Pathology, Saskatoon Health Region/University of Saskatchewan, Canada.
Rajput AH	Division of Neurology, Department of Pathology, Saskatoon Health Region/University of Saskatchewan, Canada.
South AR	cMovement Disorders Clinic, London Health Sciences Centre, 339 Windemere Blvd, A 10-026, London, Ontario Canada. asouth4@uwo.ca

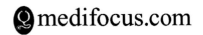

China

Name of Author	Institutional Affiliation
Jankovic J	Department of Neurology, Shanghai First People's Hospital, Shanghai Jiao Tong University School of Medicine, Shanghai, China.
Lu L	Department of Physiology, Capital Medical University, Youanmen, Beijing, PR China.
Wang X	Department of Physiology, Capital Medical University, Youanmen, Beijing, PR China.
Wu Y	Department of Neurology, Shanghai First People's Hospital, Shanghai Jiao Tong University School of Medicine, Shanghai, China.

Denmark

Name of Author	Institutional Affiliation
Olsen JH	Institute of Cancer Epidemiology, Danish Cancer Society, Strandboulevarden 49, DK-2100 Copenhagen, Denmark. rugbjerg@cancer.dk
Ritz B	Institute of Public Health, University of Copenhagen, Department of Social Medicine, Copenhagen, Denmark. n.rod@pubhealth.ku.dk
Rod NH	Institute of Public Health, University of Copenhagen, Department of Social Medicine, Copenhagen, Denmark. n.rod@pubhealth.ku.dk
Rugbjerg K	Institute of Cancer Epidemiology, Danish Cancer Society, Strandboulevarden 49, DK-2100 Copenhagen, Denmark. rugbjerg@cancer.dk

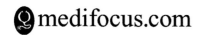

France

Name of Author	Institutional Affiliation
Bungener C	Laboratory of Clinical Psychopathology and Neuropsychology, University of Paris Descartes, Boulogne Billancourt Paris, France. montel.sebastien@wanadoo.fr
Le Jeune F	Service de Medecine Nucleaire, Centre Eugene Marquis, Renne, France.
Montel S	Laboratory of Clinical Psychopathology and Neuropsychology, University of Paris Descartes, Boulogne Billancourt Paris, France. montel.sebastien@wanadoo.fr
Rascol O	Department of Clinical Pharmacology and Neurosciences, INSERM U825 and Clinical Investigation Center, University Hospital, Toulouse, France. rascol@cict.fr
Rouaud T	Department of Neurology, University Hospital of Rennes, Rennes, France.
Verin M	Department of Neurology, University Hospital of Rennes, Rennes, France.

Germany

Name of Author	Institutional Affiliation
Botzel K	Department of Neurology, University Hospital, Ludwig-Maximilian-University, 81366 Munich, Germany. kBotzel@med.uni-muenchen.de
Chaudhuri KR	Charit Universitatsmedizin Berlin, Berlin, Germany.
Daniels C	Department of Neurology, Christian-Albrechts-University, Kiel, Germany.
Dolga AM	Institut fur Pharmakologie und Klinische Pharmazie, Philipps-Universitat Marburg, Germany.
Ebersbach G	Movement Disorders Clinic, Beelitz-Heilstatten, Germany. ebersbach@parkinson-beelitz.de
Eggert K	German Competence Network on Parkinson's Disease, Department of Neurology, Philipps-University Marburg, Marburg, Germany.

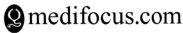
Eisel UL	Institut fur Pharmakologie und Klinische Pharmazie, Philipps-Universitat Marburg, Germany.
Hack HJ	Institute of Clinical Neuroscience and Medical Psychology, Heinrich Heine University, Universitatsstr. 1, Dusseldorf, Germany. schnitza@uni-duesseldorf.de
Kasten M	Department of Neurology, University of Lubeck, Lubeck, Germany.
Klein C	Department of Neurology, University of Lubeck, Lubeck, Germany.
Knie B	Charit Universitatsmedizin Berlin, Berlin, Germany.
Kraft E	Department of Neurology, University Hospital, Ludwig-Maximilian-University, 81366 Munich, Germany. kBotzel@med.uni-muenchen.de
Moller JC	Department of Neurology, Philipps-University, Marburg, Germany. carsten.moeller@med.uni-marburg.de
Oertel W	German Competence Network on Parkinson's Disease, Department of Neurology, Philipps-University Marburg, Marburg, Germany.
Oertel WH	Department of Neurology, Philipps-University, Marburg, Germany. carsten.moeller@med.uni-marburg.de
Schnitzler A	Institute of Clinical Neuroscience and Medical Psychology, Heinrich Heine University, Universitatsstr. 1, Dusseldorf, Germany. schnitza@uni-duesseldorf.de
Sixel-Doring F	Paracelsus-Elena-Klinik, Center of Parkinsonism and Movement Disorders, Klinikstr. 16, 34128 Kassel, Germany. friederike.sixel@pk-mx.de
Trenkwalder C	Paracelsus-Elena-Klinik, Center of Parkinsonism and Movement Disorders, Klinikstr. 16, 34128 Kassel, Germany. friederike.sixel@pk-mx.de
Wissel J	Movement Disorders Clinic, Beelitz-Heilstatten, Germany. ebersbach@parkinson-beelitz.de
Witt K	Department of Neurology, Christian-Albrechts-University, Kiel, Germany.

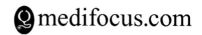

Hong Kong

Name of Author	Institutional Affiliation
Mak MK	Department of Rehabilitation Sciences, The Hong Kong Polytechnic University, Hung Hom, Hong Kong. rsmmak@inet.polyu.edu.hk
Pai YC	Department of Rehabilitation Sciences, The Hong Kong Polytechnic University, Hung Hom, Hong Kong. rsmmak@inet.polyu.edu.hk

India

Name of Author	Institutional Affiliation
Ali J	Department of Pharmaceutics, Faculty of Pharmacy, Jamia Hamdard, Hamdard Nagar, New Delhi 110062, India.
Md S	Department of Pharmaceutics, Faculty of Pharmacy, Jamia Hamdard, Hamdard Nagar, New Delhi 110062, India.
Rao VR	Anthropological Survey of India, Jawaharlal Nehru Road, India.
Sanyal J	Anthropological Survey of India, Jawaharlal Nehru Road, India.
Totey SM	Advanced Neuroscience Institute, BGS-Global Hospital, Bangalore, India. drnkvr@gmail.com
Venkataramana NK	Advanced Neuroscience Institute, BGS-Global Hospital, Bangalore, India. drnkvr@gmail.com

Israel

Name of Author	Institutional Affiliation
Hausdorff JM	Movement Disorders Unit, Department of Neurology, Tel Aviv Sourasky Medical Center, Israel. anatmi@tasmc.health.gov.il
Mirelman A	Movement Disorders Unit, Department of Neurology, Tel Aviv Sourasky Medical Center, Israel. anatmi@tasmc.health.gov.il

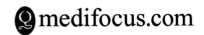

Italy

Name of Author	Institutional Affiliation
Abbruzzese G	Department for Parkinson Disease, IRCCS San Camillo, Venice, Italy. angelo3000@yahoo.com
Albanese A	Istituto di Neurologia, Universita Cattolica del Sacro Cuore, Rome, Italy.
Antonini A	IRRCS, San Camillo, Viale Alberoni 70, Venice, Italy. angelo3000@yahoo.com
Barone P	Department of Neurological Sciences, University of Napoli Federico II-IDC Hermitage Capodimonte, Naples, Italy. barone@unina.it
Berardelli A	Department of Urology and Andrology, Ospedale Santa Maria della Misericordia, University of Perugia, Perugia, Italy. agianton@libero.it
Bxarone P	Department of Neurological Sciences, University of Naples Federico II and IDC Hermitage Capodimonte, Naples, Italy. barone@unina.it
Elia AE	Fondazione, IRCCS Istituto Neurologico Carlo Besta, Universita Cattolica del Sacro Cuore, Via G. Celoria 11, 20133 Milano, Italy.
Fasano A	Istituto di Neurologia, Universita Cattolica del Sacro Cuore, Rome, Italy.
Giannantoni A	Department of Urology and Andrology, Ospedale Santa Maria della Misericordia, University of Perugia, Perugia, Italy. agianton@libero.it
Koch G	Laboratorio di Neurologia Clinica e Comportamentale Fondazione Santa Lucia, IRCCS Via Ardeatina 306 00179 Roma, Italy. g.koch@hsantalucia.it
Lopiano L	Department of Neuroscience, University of Torino, Via Cherasco 15, 10126 Turin, Italy. aristidemerola@hotmail.com
Merola A	Department of Neuroscience, University of Torino, Via Cherasco 15, 10126 Turin, Italy. aristidemerola@hotmail.com

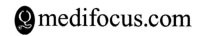
Obeso JA	Department of Neuroscience, Institute of Neurology, IRCCS San Raffaele Pisana, Roma, Italy. fabrizio.stocchi@fastwebnet.it
Odin P	IRRCS, San Camillo, Viale Alberoni 70, Venice, Italy. angelo3000@yahoo.com
Olanow CW	Institute of Neurology, IRCCS San Raffaele Pisana, Rome, Italy.
Onofrj M	Department of Neurology, University G. d'Annunzio, Chieti and Pescara, Italy.
Stanzione P	Laboratorio di Neurologia Clinica e Comportamentale Fondazione Santa Lucia, IRCCS Via Ardeatina 306 00179 Roma, Italy. g.koch@hsantalucia.it
Stocchi F	Institute of Neurology, IRCCS San Raffaele Pisana, Rome, Italy.
Thomas A	Department of Neurology, University G. d'Annunzio, Chieti and Pescara, Italy.
Weintraub D	Department of Neurological Sciences, University of Naples Federico II and IDC Hermitage Capodimonte, Naples, Italy. barone@unina.it

Japan

Name of Author	**Institutional Affiliation**
Honda Y	Department of Neurology, Mitate Hospital, Tagawa, Japan.
Inoue T	Department of Psychiatry, Hokkaido University Graduate School of Medicine, Kita-ku, Sapporo 060-8638, Japan. tinoue@med.hokudai.ac.jp
Kishi M	Neurology Division, Department of Internal Medicine, Sakura Medical Center, Toho University, Shimoshizu, Sakura 285-8741, Japan. sakakibara@sakura.med.toho-u.ac.jp
Kodama M	Department of Rehabilitation Medicine, Tokai University School of Medicine, Isehara, Kanagawa, Japan.
Koyama T	Department of Psychiatry, Hokkaido University Graduate School of Medicine, Kita-ku, Sapporo 060-8638, Japan. tinoue@med.hokudai.ac.jp

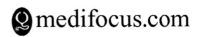

Masakado Y	Department of Rehabilitation Medicine, Tokai University School of Medicine, Isehara, Kanagawa, Japan.
Mizuno Y	Department of Neurology, Research Institute for Diseases of Old Age, Juntendo University School of Medicine, Tokyo, Japan. y_mizuno@juntendo.ac.jp
Murakami K	Department of Social and Preventive Epidemiology, School of Public Health, University of Tokyo, Hongo 7-3-1, Bunkyo-ku, Tokyo 113-0033, Japan. kenmrkm@m.u-tokyo.ac.jp
Muramatsu S	Division of Neurology, Department of Medicine, Jichi Medical University, Tochigi, Japan. muramats@jichi.ac.jp
Murata M	Department of Neurology, National Center Hospital, National Center of Neurology and Psychiatry, Kodaira, Tokyo, Japan. mihom@ncnp.go.jp
Nagai M	Department of Social and Preventive Epidemiology, School of Public Health, University of Tokyo, Hongo 7-3-1, Bunkyo-ku, Tokyo 113-0033, Japan. kenmrkm@m.u-tokyo.ac.jp
Nakano I	Division of Neurology, Department of Medicine, Jichi Medical University, Tochigi, Japan. muramats@jichi.ac.jp
Ohno Y	Laboratory of Pharmacology, Osaka University of Pharmaceutical Sciences, Nasahara, Takatsuki, Osaka, Japan. yohno@gly.oups.ac.jp
Okubo Y	Department of Neuropsychiatry, Nippon Medical School, Tokyo, Japan. sat333@nms.ac.jp
Sakakibara R	Neurology Division, Department of Internal Medicine, Sakura Medical Center, Toho University, Shimoshizu, Sakura 285-8741, Japan. sakakibara@sakura.med.toho-u.ac.jp
Sasaki T	Department of Neurosurgery, Kyushu University, Higashi-ku, Fukuoka, Japan.
Sato Y	Department of Neurology, Mitate Hospital, Tagawa, Japan.
Ueda S	Department of Neuropsychiatry, Nippon Medical School, Tokyo, Japan. sat333@nms.ac.jp

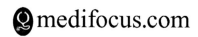

Umemura A	Department of Neurosurgery, Nagoya City University Graduate School of Medicine, 1 Kawasumi, Mizuho-ku, Nagoya 467-8601, Japan. aume@med.nagoya-cu.ac.jp
Yamada K	Department of Neurosurgery, Nagoya City University Graduate School of Medicine, 1 Kawasumi, Mizuho-ku, Nagoya 467-8601, Japan. aume@med.nagoya-cu.ac.jp
Yamamoto M	Department of Neurology, Research Institute for Diseases of Old Age, Juntendo University School of Medicine, Tokyo, Japan. y_mizuno@juntendo.ac.jp
Yoshida F	Department of Neurosurgery, Kyushu University, Higashi-ku, Fukuoka, Japan.

Korea

Name of Author	Institutional Affiliation
Hwang S	Department of Physical Therapy, College of Health Science and Social Welfare, Sahmyook University, Seoul, Korea.
Lee KS	Department of Physical Therapy, College of Health Science and Social Welfare, Sahmyook University, Seoul, Korea.

Netherlands

Name of Author	Institutional Affiliation
Esselink RA	Departments of Neurology and Geriatrics, Radboud University Nijmegen Medical Centre, Donders Institute for Brain, Cognition, and Behaviour, PO Box 9101, 6500 HB Nijmegen, the Netherlands. r.esselink@neuro.umcn.nl
Leentjens AF	Department of Psychiatry, Maastricht University Medical Centre, Maastricht, the Netherlands. a.leentjens@maastrichtuniversity.nl
Speelman JD	Departments of Neurology and Geriatrics, Radboud University Nijmegen Medical Centre, Donders Institute for Brain, Cognition, and Behaviour, PO Box 9101, 6500 HB Nijmegen, the Netherlands. r.esselink@neuro.umcn.nl

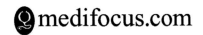

New Zealand

Name of Author	Institutional Affiliation
Anderson TJ	Van der Veer Institute for Parkinson's and Brain Research, 66 Stewart St., Christchurch 8011, New Zealand. john.dalrymple-alford@canterbury.ac.nz
Chwieduk CM	Adis, a Wolters Kluwer Business, North Shore, Auckland, New Zealand. demail@adis.co.nz
Curran MP	Adis, a Wolters Kluwer Business, North Shore, Auckland, New Zealand. demail@adis.co.nz
Dalrymple-Alford JC	Van der Veer Institute for Parkinson's and Brain Research, 66 Stewart St., Christchurch 8011, New Zealand. john.dalrymple-alford@canterbury.ac.nz
Snow BJ	Neurology Department, Auckland Hospital, Auckland, New Zealand. bsnow@adhb.govt.nz
Taylor KM	Neurology Department, Auckland Hospital, Auckland, New Zealand. bsnow@adhb.govt.nz

Norway

Name of Author	Institutional Affiliation
Aarsland D	Stavanger University Hospital, Psychiatric Division, PO Box 8100, 4068 Stavanger, Norway. daarsland@gmail.com
Alves G	The Norwegian Centre for Movement Disorders, Stavanger University Hospital, Box 8100, N-4068 Stavanger, Norway.
Emre M	Stavanger University Hospital, Psychiatric Division, PO Box 8100, 4068 Stavanger, Norway. daarsland@gmail.com
Forsaa EB	The Norwegian Centre for Movement Disorders, Stavanger University Hospital, Box 8100, N-4068 Stavanger, Norway.

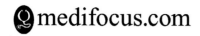

Spain

Name of Author	Institutional Affiliation
Arias P	Neuroscience and Motor Control Group (NEUROcom), Department of Medicine-INEF and Institute for Biomedical Research (INIBIC), University of A Coruna, Spain.
Cano-de-la-Cuerda R	Department of Physical Therapy, Occupational Therapy, Physical Medicine and Rehabilitation, Universidad Rey Juan Carlos, Alcorcon, Madrid, Spain.
Cudeiro J	Neuroscience and Motor Control Group (NEUROcom), Department of Physical Therapy, University of A Coruna, A Coruna, Spain.
Fernandez-de-Las-Penas C	Department of Physical Therapy, Occupational Therapy, Physical Medicine and Rehabilitation, Universidad Rey Juan Carlos, Alcorcon, Madrid, Spain.
Kulisevsky J	Unit of Movement Disorders, Neurology Department, Hospital de la Santa Creu i Sant Pau, Barcelona, Spain.
Moreno-Lopez C	Movement Disorders Unit, Department of Neurology, Hospital Clinic of Barcelona, University of Barcelona Medical School and Centro de Investigacion Biomedica en Red sobre Enfermedades Neurodegenerativas, 08036 Barcelona, Spain.
Pagonabarraga J	Unit of Movement Disorders, Neurology Department, Hospital de la Santa Creu i Sant Pau, Barcelona, Spain.
Tolosa E	Movement Disorders Unit, Department of Neurology, Hospital Clinic of Barcelona, University of Barcelona Medical School and Centro de Investigacion Biomedica en Red sobre Enfermedades Neurodegenerativas, 08036 Barcelona, Spain.
Vivas J	Neuroscience and Motor Control Group (NEUROcom), Department of Physical Therapy, University of A Coruna, A Coruna, Spain.

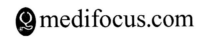

Sweden

Name of Author	Institutional Affiliation
Hamberg K	Department of Community Medicine and Rehabilitation, Occupational Therapy, University of Umea, Sweden. gun-marie.hariz@neuro.umu.se
Hariz GM	Department of Community Medicine and Rehabilitation, Occupational Therapy, University of Umea, Sweden. gun-marie.hariz@neuro.umu.se
Lokk J	Institution of Neurobiology, Care Sciences and Society, Karolinska Institutet, Geriatric Dept, Karolinska University Hospital Huddinge, SE-14186 Stockholm, Sweden. johan.lokk@karolinska.se
Nilsson M	Institution of Neurobiology, Care Sciences and Society, Karolinska Institutet, Geriatric Dept, Karolinska University Hospital Huddinge, SE-14186 Stockholm, Sweden. johan.lokk@karolinska.se

Switzerland

Name of Author	Institutional Affiliation
Benninger DH	Department of Neurology, University Hospital of Basel, Petersgraben 4, 4051 Basel, Switzerland. benningerd@uhbs.ch
Hallett M	Department of Neurology, University Hospital of Basel, Petersgraben 4, 4051 Basel, Switzerland. benningerd@uhbs.ch
Kaelin-Lang A	Movement Disorders Center, Department of Neurology, "Inselspital" Berne University Hospital, University of Berne, Switzerland.
Kipfer S	Movement Disorders Center, Department of Neurology, "Inselspital" Berne University Hospital, University of Berne, Switzerland.

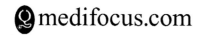

Turkey

Name of Author	Institutional Affiliation
Emre M	Istanbul University, Istanbul Faculty of Medicine, Istanbul, Turkey. muratemre@superonline.com
Erginoz E	Department of Neurology, Sisli Etfal Education and Research Hospital, Istanbul, Turkey.
Jones R	Istanbul University, Istanbul Faculty of Medicine, Istanbul, Turkey. muratemre@superonline.com
Kenangil G	Department of Neurology, Sisli Etfal Education and Research Hospital, Istanbul, Turkey.
Kulaksizoglu H	Selcuk University, Selcuklu Medical School, Department of Urology, Turkey. kulaksizoglu@superonline.com
Parman Y	Selcuk University, Selcuklu Medical School, Department of Urology, Turkey. kulaksizoglu@superonline.com

United Kingdom

Name of Author	Institutional Affiliation
Barker RA	Cambridge Centre for Brain Repair, Department of Clinical Neurosciences, University of Cambridge, Forvie Site, Robinson Way, Cambridge, CB2 0PY, UK. chm27@cam.ac.uk
Berry AL	Department of Molecular Neuroscience, UCL Institute of Neurology, Queen Square, London, WC1N 3BG, UK.
Burn DJ	Institute for Ageing and Health, Newcastle University, Newcastle upon Tyne, UK.
Chaudhuri KR	Guy's, King's & St Thomas' School of Medicine, King's College, London, UK.
Docherty MJ	Institute for Ageing and Health, Newcastle University, Newcastle upon Tyne, UK.
Foltynie T	UCL Institute of Neurology, Queen Square, London, UK. t.foltynie@ion.ucl.ac.uk
Furmston A	Birmingham Clinical Trials Unit, University of Birmingham, Edgbaston, Birmingham, UK, B15 2TT.

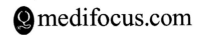

Hallett M	Behavioural and Clinical Neurosciences Institute, Department of Experimental Psychology, Downing Site, University of Cambridge, Cambridge CB2 3EB, UK. vv247@cam.ac.uk
Hamdy S	University of Manchester, Salford, UK.
Haq IZ	Guy's, King's & St Thomas' School of Medicine, King's College, London, UK.
Hariz MI	UCL Institute of Neurology, Queen Square, London, UK. t.foltynie@ion.ucl.ac.uk
Hobson P	Academic Unit (North Wales), Cardiff University, Glan Clwyd Hospital, Rhyl, UK. peterhobson@hotmail.com
Ishihara-Paul L	Academic Unit (North Wales), Cardiff University, Glan Clwyd Hospital, Rhyl, UK. peterhobson@hotmail.com
Johns C	University of Bedfordshire, Putteridge Bury, Hitchin Road, Luton, LU2 8LE, UK. chris.johns@beds.ac.uk
Lees AJ	Queen Square Brain Bank for Neurological Disorders, UCL Institute of Neurology, UK.
Limousin P	Sobell Department, Unit of Functional Neurosurgery, UCL Institute of Neurology, Box 146, Queen Square, London, WC1N 3BG, UK. e.tripoliti@ion.ucl.ac.uk
Linazasoro G	Consultant Physician and Honorary Professor, Sherwood Forest hospitals NHS Trust, University of Nottingham, UK. jagsharma@tiscali.co.uk
Michou E	University of Manchester, Salford, UK.
Parkkinen L	Queen Square Brain Bank for Neurological Disorders, UCL Institute of Neurology, UK.
Pennington S	ST3 Palliative Medicine Marie Curie hospice, Marie Curie Drive, Newcastle upon Tyne, UK.
Piccini P	Department of Clinical Neurosciences, Faculty of Medicine, Hammersmith Hospital, Imperial College, London, United Kingdom. marios.politis@imperial.ac.uk
Poewe W	Institute of Neurology, University College London, London, UK. a.schapira@ucl.ac.uk

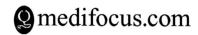
Politis M	Department of Clinical Neurosciences, Faculty of Medicine, Hammersmith Hospital, Imperial College, London, United Kingdom. marios.politis@imperial.ac.uk
Revesz T	Department of Molecular Neuroscience and Reta Lila Weston Institute of Neurological Studies, Institute of Neurology, University College London and the National Hospital for Neurology and Neurosurgery, London, UK. alees@ion.ucl.ac.uk
Schapira AH	Institute of Neurology, University College London, London, UK. a.schapira@ucl.ac.uk
Sharma JC	Consultant Physician and Honorary Professor, Sherwood Forest hospitals NHS Trust, University of Nottingham, UK. jagsharma@tiscali.co.uk
Sinclair A	University of Bedfordshire, Putteridge Bury, Hitchin Road, Luton, LU2 8LE, UK. chris.johns@beds.ac.uk
Stowe R	Birmingham Clinical Trials Unit, University of Birmingham, Edgbaston, Birmingham, UK, B15 2TT.
Tripoliti E	Sobell Department, Unit of Functional Neurosurgery, UCL Institute of Neurology, Box 146, Queen Square, London, WC1N 3BG, UK. e.tripoliti@ion.ucl.ac.uk
Voon V	Behavioural and Clinical Neurosciences Institute, Department of Experimental Psychology, Downing Site, University of Cambridge, Cambridge CB2 3EB, UK. vv247@cam.ac.uk
Walker R	ST3 Palliative Medicine Marie Curie hospice, Marie Curie Drive, Newcastle upon Tyne, UK.
Wheatley K	Queen Elizabeth Hospital, Birmingham, Birmingham, UK.
Williams A	Queen Elizabeth Hospital, Birmingham, Birmingham, UK.
Williams-Gray CH	Cambridge Centre for Brain Repair, Department of Clinical Neurosciences, University of Cambridge, Forvie Site, Robinson Way, Cambridge, CB2 0PY, UK. chm27@cam.ac.uk

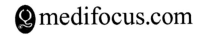

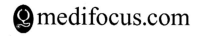

NOTES

Use this page for taking notes as you review your Guidebook

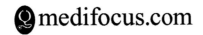

5 - Tips on Finding and Choosing a Doctor

Introduction

One of the most important decisions confronting patients who have been diagnosed with a serious medical condition is finding and choosing a qualified physician who will deliver a high level and quality of medical care in accordance with currently accepted guidelines and standards of care. Finding the "best" doctor to manage your condition, however, can be a frustrating and time-consuming experience unless you know what you are looking for and how to go about finding it.

The process of finding and choosing a physician to manage your specific illness or condition is, in some respects, analogous to the process of making a decision about whether or not to invest in a particular stock or mutual fund. After all, you wouldn't invest your hard eared money in a stock or mutual fund without first doing exhaustive research about the stock or fund's past performance, current financial status, and projected future earnings. More than likely you would spend a considerable amount of time and energy doing your own research and consulting with your stock broker before making an informed decision about investing. The same general principle applies to the process of finding and choosing a physician. Although the process requires a considerable investment in terms of both time and energy, the potential payoff can be well worth it--after all, what can be more important than your health and well-being?

This section of your Guidebook offers important tips for how to find physicians as well as suggestions for how to make informed choices about choosing a doctor who is right for you.

Tips for Finding Physicians

Finding a highly qualified, competent, and compassionate physician to manage your specific illness or condition takes a lot of hard work and energy but is an investment that is well-worth the effort. It is important to keep in mind that you are not looking for just any general physician but rather for a physician who has expertise in the treatment and management of your specific illness or condition. Here are some suggestions for where you can turn to identify and locate physicians who specialize in managing your disorder:

medifocus.com

- **Your Doctor** - Your family physician (family medicine or internal medicine specialist) is a good starting point for finding a physician who specializes in your illness. Chances are that your doctor already knows several specialists in your geographic area who specialize in your illness and can recommend several names to you. Your doctor can also provide you with information about their qualifications, training, and hospital affiliations.

- **Your Peer Network** - Your family, friends, and co-workers can be a potentially very useful network for helping you find a physician who specializes in your illness. They may know someone else with this condition and may be able to put you in touch with them to find out which doctors they can recommend. If you have friends, neighbors, or relatives who work in hospitals (e.g., nurses, social workers, administrators), they may be a potentially valuable source for helping you find a physician who specializes in your condition.

- **Hospitals and Medical Centers** - Hospitals and medical centers are, potentially, an excellent source for finding physicians who specialize in treating specific diseases. Simply contact hospitals and major medical centers in your city, county, or state and ask if they have anyone on their staff who specializes in treating your condition. When you call, ask to speak to someone in the specific Department that cares for patients with the illness. For example, if you have been diagnosed with cancer, ask to speak with someone in the Department of Hematology and Oncology. If you are not sure which Department treats patients with your specific condition, ask to speak to someone in the Department of Medicine since this Department is the umbrella for many other medical specialties.

- **Organizations and Support Groups** - Many disease organizations and support groups that cater to patients with a specific illness or condition maintain physician referral lists and may be able to recommend doctors in your geographic area who specialize in the treatment and management of your specific disorder. This *MediFocus Guidebook* includes a select listing of disease organizations and support groups that you may wish to contact to ask for a physician referral.

- **Managed Care Plans** - If you belong to a managed care plan, you can obtain a list of physicians who belong to the Plan from the plan's membership services office. Keep in mind, however, that your choices will usually be limited to only those doctors who belong to the Plan. If you decide to go outside the Plan, you will likely have to pay for the doctor's services "out of pocket".

- **Medical Journals** - Many doctors based at major medical centers and universities who have special interest in a particular disease or condition conduct research and publish their findings in leading medical journals. Searching the medical literature can help you identify and locate leading physicians who are recognized as experts in their field about a particular illness. This *MediFocus Guidebook* includes an extensive listing of the names and institutional affiliations of physicians and researchers, in the United States and other countries, who have recently published their studies about this specific medical condition in leading medical journals. You can also conduct your own online search for your illness or condition and identify additional authors and hospitals who specialize in the disease using the PubMed database available at http://www.nlm.nih.gov.

- **American Medical Association** - The American Medical Association (AMA) is the nation's largest professional medical association that represents many doctors in the United States and also provides a free physician locator service called "AMA Physician Select" available at http://dbapps.ama-assn.org/aps/amahg.htm. You can search the AMA database by either "Physician Name" or "Medical Specialty". You can find information about physicians including medical school and residency training, area of specialty, and contact information.

- **American Board of Medical Specialists** - The American Board of Medical Specialists (ABMS) publishes a geographical list of board-certified physicians called the Official ABMS Directory of Board Certified Medical Specialists that is available in most public libraries. Physicians who are listed in the ABMS Directory are board-certified in a medical specialty meaning that they have passed rigorous certification examinations administered by a board of medical specialists. There are 24 specialty boards that are recognized by the ABMS and the AMA. Each candidate applying for board certification must pass a written examination given by the specific specialty board and 15 of the specialty boards also require candidates to pass an oral examination in order to obtain board certification. To find out if a particular physician you are considering is board certified:

  - Visit your local public library and ask for a copy of the Official ABMS Directory of Board Certified Medical Specialists.

  - Search the ABMS web site at http://www.abms.org/login.asp.

  - Call the ABMS toll free at 1-866-275-2267.

- **American Society of Clinical Oncology** - The American Society of Clinical Onclology (ASC)) is the largest professional organization that represents physicians who specialize in treating cancer patients (oncologists). The ASCO provides a searchable database of ASCO members called "Find an Oncologist" that you can access online at http://www.asco.org. You can search the "Find an Oncologist" database for a cancer specialist by name, city, state, country, or specialty area.

- **American Cancer Society** - The American Cancer Society (ACS) is a nationwide voluntary health organization dedicated to helping cancer patients and survivors through research, education, advocacy, and services. The ACS web site http://www.cancer.org is not only an excellent resource for cancer information but also includes a "Message Board" where you can ask questions, exchange ideas, and share stories. The ACS Message Board is also a potentially useful source for locating an oncologist in your geographical area who specializes in your specific type of cancer. You can also contact the ACS toll free by calling 1-800-ACS-2345.

- **National Comprehensive Cancer Network** - The National Comprehensive Cancer Network (NCCN) is an alliance of 19 of the world's leading cancer centers and is dedicated to helping patients and health care professionals make informed decisions about cancer care. You can find a listing of the 19 NCCN member cancer institutions on the NCCN web site at http://www.nccn.org/. You can also search the NCCN "Physician Directory" for doctors located at any of the 19 NCCN member cancer institutions at http://www.nccn.org/physician_directory/SearchPers.asp. This database is an excellent resource for locating leading cancer specialists nationwide who specialize in your specific type of cancer.

- **National Cancer Institute Clinical Trials Database** - The National Cancer Institute (NCI) is part of the National Institutes of Health (NIH) and coordinates the National Cancer Program which conducts and supports research, training, and a variety of other programs dedicated to prevention and treatment of cancer. The NCI maintains an extensive cancer clinical trials database that you can access at http://www.cancer.gov/clinicaltrials. You can search the database for current clinical trials by type of cancer and even limit your search to clinical trials within you geographical area by putting in your Zip Code. The NCI clinical trials database also provides contact information for the physicians who serve as the study coordinators for each clinical trial. This database is a valuable resource for identifying and locating leading physicians in your local area and around the country who are conducting cutting-edge clinical research about your specific type of cancer.

- **National Center for Complementary and Alternative Medicine** - The National Center for Complementary and Alternative Medicine (NCCAM) is part of the National Institutes of Health (NIH) and is dedicated to exploring complementary and alternative medicine healing practices in the context of rigorous scientific research and methodology. The NCCAM web site http://nccam.nih.gov/ includes publications, frequently asked questions, and useful links to other complementary and alternative medicine resources. If you have questions about complementary and alternative medicine practices for your particular illness or medical condition, you can contact

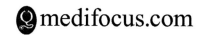

the NCCAM Clearinghouse toll-free in the U.S. at 1-888-644-6226 or 301-519-3153. You can also contact the NCCAM Clearinghouse by E-mail: info@nccam.nih.gov.

- **National Organization for Rare Disorders** - The National Organization for Rare Disorders (NORD) is a federation of voluntary health organizations dedicated to helping patients with rare "orphan" diseases and their families. There are over 6,000 rare or "orphan" diseases that are estimated to affect approximately 25 million Americans. You can search NORD's "Rare Diseases Database" for information about rare diseases at http://www.rarediseases.org/search/rdblist.html. In addition to providing useful information about rare diseases, NORD maintains a confidential "Networking Program" for its members to enable them to communicate with other patients who suffer from the same disorder. To learn more about NORD's Networking Program, you can send an E mail to: orphan@rarediseases.org.

How to Make Informed Choices About Physicians

It has generally been assumed by many people that the longer a physician has been in practice, the more experience, knowledge, and skills he/she has accumulated and, therefore, the higher the quality of care they provide to their patients. Recent research conducted by a group of doctors from the Harvard Medical School, however, seems to strongly suggest that this premise may not be true. In an article published in February 2005 in the *Annals of Internal Medicine* (Volume 142, No. 4, pp. 260-303), the Harvard researchers seriously challenged the common assumption that the more clinical experience a physician has accumulated, the higher the level of medical care they provide to their patients.

In fact, surprisingly, the researchers found an inverse (opposite) relationship between the number of years that a physician has been in practice (i.e., experience) and the quality of care that the physician provides. In other words, the widely held belief that "practice makes perfect" does not necessarily apply to all physicians and should not be the sole criteria used by patients in their decision analysis for choosing a physician. The underlying message of this study is that the length of time a physician has been in practice does not necessarily equate to a high quality of medical care unless the doctor takes steps to keep abreast with new advances and changing patterns of clinical practice.

Here are some important issues you need to consider and carefully research before making an informed decision about choosing your doctor:

- **Board Certification** - Board certified doctors are required to have extra training after medical school to become specialists in a particular field of medicine and are required to take continuing education courses in order to maintain their board certification status. Check with the American Board of Medical Specialists (ABMS) to determine if a specific physician you are considering is board certified in a particular medical specialty. To find out if a particular physician you are considering is board certified:

  - Visit your local public library and ask for a copy of the Official ABMS Directory of Board Certified Medical Specialists.

  - Search the ABMS web site at http://www.abms.org/login.asp.

  - Call the ABMS toll free at 1-866-275-2267.

- **Experience** - As noted above, research from the Harvard Medical School strongly suggests that how long a physician has been in practice (i.e., experience) does not necessarily correlate with a high level of medical care. The most important issue, therefore, is not how long a doctor has been in practice but rather how much experience the physician has in treating your specific illness or medical condition. Some physicians who have been in practice for many decades may have only treated a small number of patients with the specific disorder, whereas, some younger physicians who have been in practice only a few years may have already treated hundreds of patients with the same disorder. Here are some suggestions for helping you find out about a particular physician's experience in treating your specific illness:

  - Call the physician's office and speak with a staff member such as a nurse or physician's assistant. Ask them for information about how many patients with your specific medical condition the physician treats during the course of a year. Ask how many patients with this condition the physician is currently treating. You will have to call several different physicians' offices in order to have a basis for comparing the numbers of patients.

  - Find out if the physician has published any articles about the condition in reputable medical journals by doing an author search online. You can conduct an online author search using PubMed at http://www.nlm.nih.gov. Simply click on the "PubMed" icon, select the "author" field from the "Limits" menu, enter the physician's name (last name followed by first initial), and then click on the "Go" button. The author search will retrieve all articles published by the particular physician you are considering.

- Talk with your family physician and ask if he/she can provide you with any information about the particular physician's experience in treating patients with your specific illness or condition.

- Contact disease organizations and support groups that specialize in helping patients with your specific disorder and ask if they can provide you with any information, including experience, about the physician you are considering.

- **Medical School Affiliation** - Find out if the physician you are considering also has a joint faculty appointment at a medical school. In general, practicing community physicians with a joint academic appointment at a medical school are more likely to be in contact with leading medical experts and may be more up-to-date with the latest advances in research and treatments than community based physicians who are not affiliated with a medical school.

- **Hospital Affiliation** - Find out about the hospitals that the doctor uses. In the event that you need to be treated at a hospital, is the hospital where the physician has admitting privileges nearby to your home or will you (and your family members) have to travel a considerable distance?

- **Hospital Accreditation** - Find out if the hospital where the physician has admitting privileges is accredited by the Joint Commission on Accreditation of Healthcare Organizations (JCAHO). You can find information about a specific hospital's accreditation status by searching the JCAHO web site at http://www.jointcommission.org/. The JCAHO is an independent, not-for-profit organization that evaluates and accredits more than 15,000 health care organizations and programs in the United States. To receive and maintain JCAHO accreditation, a health care organization must undergo an on-site survey by a JCAHO survey team at least every three years and meet specific standards and performance measurements that affect the safety and quality of patient care.

- **Health Insurance Coverage** - Find out if the physician is covered by your health insurance plan. If you belong to a managed care plan (HMO or PPO), you are usually restricted to using specific physicians who also belong to the Plan. If you decide to use a physician who is "outside the network," you will likely have to pay "out of pocket" for the services provided.

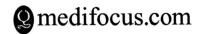

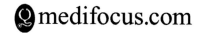

NOTES

Use this page for taking notes as you review your Guidebook

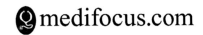

6 - Directory of Organizations

American Academy of Neurology
1080 Montreal Avenue; St. Paul, MN 55116
800.879.1960   651.695.2717
memberservies@aan.com
www.aan.com

American Association of Neurological Surgeons
5550 Meadowbrook Drive; Rolling Meadows, IL 60088
888.566.AANS 847.378-0500; 847.378.0600 (fax)
info@aans.org
www.neurosurgery.org

American Parkinson Disease Association
135 Parkinson Avenue; Staten Island, NY 10305
718.981.8001; 800.223.2732
apda@apdaparkinson.org
www.apdaparkinson.org

Bachmann-Strauss Dystonia & Parkinsons Disease Foundation
Mt. Sinai Medical Center; Fred French Building 551 5th Avenue Suite 520 New York,
NY 10176
212.682.9900
www.dystonia-parkinsons.org

Cure Parkinson's Trust; Movers and Shakers
The VEstry 1 St. Clement\'s Court London EC4N 7HB UK
020 7929 7656
info@cureparkinsons.org.uk
www.cureparkinsons.org.uk

European Parkinsons Disease Association
4 Golding Road; Sevenoaks, Kent; TN13 3NJ UNITED KINGDOM
44(0) 1732 457 683
lizzie@epda.eu.com
www.epda.eu.com

Family Caregiver Alliance
180 Montgomery Street; Suite 1100; San Francisco, CA 94104
800.445.8106   415.434.3388
info@caregiver.org
www.caregiver.org

Michael J. Fox Foundation for Parkinson's Research
Church Street Station Box 780 New York, NY 10008
800.708.7644
michaeljfox.org

National Family Caregivers Association (NFCA)
10400 Connecticut Avenue; #500; Kensington, MD 20895-3944
800.896.3650 301.942.6430; 301.942.2302 (f)
info@nfcacares.org
www.nfcacares.org

National Institute of Neurological Disorders and Stroke
P.O. Box 5801; Bethesda, MD 20842
800.352.9424   301.496.5751; 301.468.5981 (TTY)
www.ninds.nih.gov

National Parkinson Foundation
1501 NW Ninth Avenue/Bob Hope Road; Miami, FL 33136-9990
800.327.4545   305.243.6666; 305.243.5595 (fax)
contact@parkinson.org
www.parkinson.org

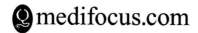

National Young Onset Center

Glenbrook Hospital 2100 Pfingsten Road; Glenview, IL 60026
877.223.3801
apda@youngparkinsons.org
www.youngparkinsons.org

Parkinson's Disease Foundation

1359 Broadway; Suite 1509; New York, NY 10018
800.457.6676 212.923.4700; 212.923.4778 (fax)
info@pdf.org
www.pdf.org

Parkinson's Disease Society of the UK

215 Vauxhall Bridge Road; London SW1V 1EJ; UNITED KINGDOM
020 7931 8080   0808 800 0303 (helpline)
enquiries@parkinsons.org.uk
www.parkinsons.org.uk

Parkinsons Society of Canada

4211 Yonge Street; Suite 316; Toronto, M2P 2A9 CANADA
800.565.3000   416.227.9700; 416.227.9600 (fax)
general.info@parkinson.ca
www.parkinson.ca

Parkinson's Action Network (PAN)

1025 Vermont Avenue NW; Suite 1120; Washington, DC 20005
800.850.4726; 202.638.4104
info@parkinsonsaction.org
www.parkinsonsaction.org

Parkinson's Resource Organization

74090 El Passeo; Suite 102; Palm Desert, CA 92260-4135
877.775.4111; 760.773.5628
info@parkinsonsresource.org
www.parkinsonsresource.org

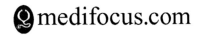medifocus.com

Parkinson's Australia

Frewin Centre Frewin Place Scullin ACT 2614
02 6278 8916
parkinsonsw@bigpond.com
www.parkinsons.org.au

Resources for Rehabilitation

22 Bonad Road; Winchester, MA 01890
781.368.9094; 718.368.9096 (fax)
info@rfr.org
www.rfr.org

The Movement Disorders Society

555 East Wells Street; Suite 1100; Milwaukee, WI 53202-3823
414.276.2145
info@movementdisorders.org
www.movementdisorders.org

The Parkinson Alliance

POB 308; Kingston, NJ 08528
800.579.8440 609.688.0870; 609.688.0875 (f)
admin@parkinsonalliance.net
www.parkinsonalliance.net

The Parkinson's Institute

675 Almanor Avenue Sunnyvale, CA 94085
800.786.2958; 800.655.2273; 408.734.2800
outreach@parkinsonsinstitute.org
www.parkinsonsinstitute.org

World Parkinsons Disease Association

via Zuretti 35 20125 Milano Italy
(39) 02.6671.3111
info@wpda.org
www.wpda.org

Worldwide Education & Awareness for Movement Disorders; (WEMOVE)

204 W. 84th Street; New York, NY 10024
800.437.6682 212.875.8312
wemove@wemove.org
www.wemove.org

Young Onset Parkinson's Association

2910 Commercial Center Blvd. Box 106 Katy, TX 77494

888.937.9672
yopaboard@yopa.org
www.yopa.org

Young Parkinson's Support Network of California; APDA Young Parkinson's I&R Center

1041 Foxenwood Drive; Santa Maria, CA 93455
800.223.9776 805.934.2216

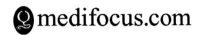

Complementary and Alternative Medicine Resources

American Academy of Medical Acupuncture

170 East Grand Avenue Suite 330 El Segundo, CA 90245 Phone: 310.364.0193
administrato@medicalacupuncture.org
http://www.medicalacupuncture.org

American Association for Acupuncture and Oriental Medicine

1925 West County Road B2
Roseville, MN 55113
Phone: 651.631.0216
http://www.aaaom.edu

American Association of Naturopathic Physicians

4435 Wisconsin Avenue
Suite 403 Washington, DC 20016
Phone (Toll free): 866.538.2267
Phone: 202.237.8150
http://www.naturopathic.org

American Chiropractic Association

1701 Clarendon Blvd.
Arlington, VA 22209
Phone: 703.276.8800 memberinfo@acatoday.org http://www.amerchiro.org

American Holistic Medical Association

23366 Commerce Park Suite 101B Beachwood, OH 44122 Phone: 216.292.6644
info@holisticmedicine.org http://www.holisticmedicine.org

American Massage Therapy Association

500 Davis Street, Suite 900
Evanston, IL 60201-4695
Phone (Toll-Free): 877.905.2700
Phone: 847.864.0123 info@amtamassage.org http://www.amtamassage.org

National Center for Complementary and Alternative Medicine (NCCAM) Clearinghouse

9000 Rockville Pike Bethesda, MD 20892 Phone: 888.644.6226 info@nccam.nih.gov

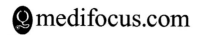

http://nccam.nih.gov

National Center for Homeopathy

801 North Fairfax Street, Suite 306
Alexandria, VA 22314
Phone: 703.548.7790
http://www.homeopathic.org

Office of Dietary Supplements, National Institutes of Health

6100 Executive Boulevard
Room 3B01, MSC 7517
Bethesda, MD 20892-7517
Phone: 301.435.2920 ods@nih.gov http://ods.od.nih.gov

Rosenthal Center for Complementary and Alternative Medicine

Columbia Presbyterian Hospital
630 West 168th Street
Box 75
New York, NY 10032
Phone: 212.342.0101
http://rosenthal.hs.columbia.edu

CPSIA information can be obtained at www.ICGtesting.com
Printed in the USA
LVOW031335170212

269185LV00001B/2/P